Based on sound dietary principles,
**SUGAR BUSTERS!®**
is a highly effective program that shows you how to
reduce sugar in your life (without feeling deprived)
through easy-to-follow recipes and meal plans.
In this new edition, you will discover

- A discussion on prevention, still the best medicine
- A special section on childhood obesity—how to
  measure it and what to to about it
- Hard facts on soft drinks
- A Body Mass Index (BMI) chart and Calculation
  Formula to determine if you are obese or merely
  overweight
- An expanded discussion of our ancestors' diet,
  which was whole-grain, high-fiber, and low
  glycemic—just like SUGAR BUSTERS!
- Handy information on how SUGAR BUSTERS!
  compares with other diet plans, from Atkins to
  Ornish

# THE NEW
# SUGAR BUSTERS!®

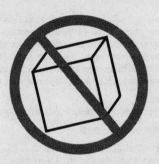

# CUT SUGAR TO TRIM FAT

*Revised and Updated*

**H. LEIGHTON STEWARD**

**MORRISON C. BETHEA, M.D.**

**SAM S. ANDREWS, M.D.**

**LUIS A. BALART, M.D.**

BALLANTINE BOOKS · NEW YORK

The information and advice presented in this book are not meant to substitute for the advice of your physician or other trained health-care professionals. You are advised to consult with health-care professionals with regard to all matters that may require medical attention or diagnosis and to check with a physician before administering or undertaking any course of treatment or diet.

A Ballantine Book
Published by The Random House Publishing Group

Copyright © 2003 by Sugar Busters LLC

www.ballantinebooks.com

ISBN 0-345-46958-5

Manufactured in the United States of America

First Ballantine Books Hardcover Edition: January 2003
First Ballantine Books Mass Market Edition: December 2003

OPM 10 9 8 7 6 5 4 3 2 1

Dedicated to all those who have improved their weight and general health, particularly diabetics, thus confirming that the diet humans consumed over the past millennia, which did not contain refined sugar or refined grains, is still the healthiest way to eat.

# Contents

# Preface

Readers may well ask why we have written a revised *Sugar Busters!* Do the recommendations for following the *Sugar Busters!* lifestyle need changing? Has the *Sugar Busters!* lifestyle turned out to be just another fad diet, as some critics asserted? Absolutely not! The lifestyle has proven to be solid, simple, successful, and most of all, healthful.

This success has created the need to add many new chapters to expand on the benefits of this way of eating and living. Eighteen key new chapters include "Prevention" (addressing weight and health problems), "The Epidemic of Childhood Obesity" (and what to do about it), "Exercise" (to further emphasize this important aspect of healthy living), "Super Foods" (to help make sure you consume some of the best of the best), "Soft Drinks, Hard Facts" (to further alert you to this growing problem), and "Calculating Fatness and Obesity" (to help determine how much you or your child is overweight).

There are also chapters to give you a more in-depth

understanding of the *Sugar Busters!* lifestyle, including "The Glycemic Index," "Reading Labels," "The Plateaus," "Stocking and Unstocking the Pantry," "Lifetime Meal Plans," "Alternative Sweeteners," "To Drink or Not to Drink," "Fat Versus Low-Fat Diets and Products," and "Why *Sugar Busters!*"

We have included recipes from well known restaurants in North America and around the world so when you travel you will know there are *Sugar Busters!*-friendly restaurants in your path.

You will also find, from the Introduction onward, references to studies performed around the world that provide verification of the benefits of the various aspects of the *Sugar Busters!* lifestyle.

Because most diets are aimed at weight loss, they have historically recommended reducing calories and/or fat; this practice is unnatural to an affluent society or even the Eskimos of North America. America is in dire need of a way of eating (and drinking) that will allow its people to consume reasonable quantities of food that can improve their daily enjoyment of life. At the same time, this new way of eating should eliminate unwanted quantities of weight and, more importantly, the adverse effects current eating habits have on blood cholesterol, triglycerides, and causing, or negatively affecting, diseases such as diabetes.

Is a diet really needed to enhance everybody's health and performance? A large percentage of our population is faced with the daily decisions and stress levels that were afforded only to some of the country's top leaders just a few decades ago. In our lives today, at home and work and in between, we are faced with constant demands; phone calls, faxes, computer problems and opportunities, high speed, close-quarter traffic situations, and dawn-to-dawn media bombardments of local and worldwide murders, pestilence, catastrophes, and wars. So, we all need to be ready to best handle the mental and physical demands each day presents and a good lifestyle is the best way to prepare for the challenges.

We authors are still excited and highly motivated to get this message out to benefit humankind—and humankind certainly is in need of some help in the area of eating habits.

One author, a former Fortune 500 CEO, is in his sixties and slim. He has been eating the way this book recommends for over nine years and is still twenty pounds down from his starting weight and has significantly improved his blood chemistry. All this at an average of over 3,100 calories a day!

Our three doctor authors include a cardiovascular surgeon, an endocrinologist, and a gastroenterologist. These are not ordinary doctors. Our heart surgeon has been voted the number-one cardiovascular surgeon in the greater New Orleans area by his peers, the most respected vote a doctor can receive. The endocrinologist is a member of the Audubon Internal Medicine Group at the largest hospital in New

Orleans. Our gastroenterologist is chief of the gastroenterology section at the Louisiana State University Health Sciences Center in New Orleans, and is an expert in liver function and metabolism and was invaluable in pointing out the connections between various hormonal secretions and the liver, where cholesterol is manufactured.

# Acknowledgments

Meaningful revisions to a way of eating that has been good for the human race for millions of years are not easy to come by. Additional documentation and explanation regarding the benefits of this lifestyle, however, can help convince some to try this way of eating, which can lead to a longer and healthier life. We therefore acknowledge those who are doing the controlled medical studies that are continuing to validate the principles in *Sugar Busters!* We believe these studies will ultimately silence those who would theorize nutritional regimens based on misguided intuitions rather than sound scientific fact.

# THE NEW
# SUGAR BUSTERS!®

# 1 | Introduction

Since *Sugar Busters! Cut Sugar to Trim Fat* was first published in 1995, confirmations of the success and wisdom of this way of eating have continued to be documented in clinical studies, testimonials, and the nutritional literature. Large numbers of doctors all over the country are not only following the *Sugar Busters!* lifestyle, but recommending it to their patients. Medical studies are proving that high-fiber, low-glycemic diets, like the *Sugar Busters!* lifestyle recommends, are good for weight control and control of many medical maladies. The low-sugar, low-glycemic, high-fiber diet helps, or in some cases even prevents, problems such as obesity, diabetes, cardiovascular diseases and many others that will be discussed later in this book.

You may have heard the statistic that obesity has risen as much in the last ten years as in the previous four decades combined. While we cannot prove or disprove these statistics, we do know that obesity is rising so rapidly that it is about to replace smoking as the number-one killer in the United States. Ten years ago, smoking killed 430,000 people a year and obesity killed 325,000 a year. Smoking-related death rates are going down, but obesity-related rates are still climbing.

Fortunately, both smoking and becoming obese are lifestyle choices. All smokers can quit, and over 90 percent of obese or overweight individuals can better control their weight with just two steps: finding a safe and easy way to accomplish that goal, and giving it a shot. Pounds cannot be "thought" off. We will tell you how to lose weight and, just as important, how to keep it off. Unlike so many diets that put you through a crash phase or deprivation phase and then an adjusted phase, the *Sugar Busters!* lifestyle gets you to "start out like you can hold out," yes, that you can maintain for the rest of your life. Since you will not be deprived of normal amounts of foods, this will be much easier than you might imagine.

What is the secret that makes the *Sugar Busters!* lifestyle so simple, easy, effective, and inexpensive? Let us boil all this down to its essence in one sentence: We are recommending that you eat like your ancestors ate (until very recently), because they ate zero refined sugar and only whole-grain and unrefined foods. That is what Mother Nature provided. That is the eating plan that got us here. It was a high-fiber, low-glycemic diet that contained no refined sugar (see Chapter 10). A little honey was available for the chiefs or royalty, or for those who braved the bees, but not for the general population of the time. Sugar and the sweet tastes of the day came from natural fruits and vegetables.

What do anthropologists tell us about these ancestors of ours? They tell us that obesity, diabetes, and heart disease appear to have been quite rare.

Remember that the number-two killer (soon to be number one) at the dawn of the twenty-first century is obesity. What two diseases are strongly associated with obesity? You are right: diabetes and heart disease. To further get you in the mood to absorb the way of eating recommended in this book, think about the following. Dr. Thomas Farley, chairman of the Department of Community Health Sciences at Tulane University's School of Public Health and Tropical Medicine, recently wrote that in the forty years between 1958 and 1998, the number of Americans diagnosed with diabetes rose 600 percent! Of course, more people are being screened for diabetes today, but the increase in diabetes is still tremendous. According to the government, diabetes alone is costing the United States over $44 billion a year. That is hundreds of dollars apiece for the average taxpayer to treat something that, as you will see, is largely preventable.

In addition to diabetes, obesity can cause you who

are obese *and your obese children* the following problems: heart disease, high blood pressure, stroke, kidney failure, cancer (colon, breast, and prostate), gallstones, poor circulation (amputations), arthritis, pregnancy complications, menstrual irregularities, stress, incontinence, and depression. Diabetes can also lead to blindness.

Thirty years ago, following the 1972 Olympics, the country went on a fitness kick, and a larger percent of the population started exercising. This lasted about a decade. In that same decade, we were advised to shift to a low-fat, high-carbohydrate diet. We did, and the rate of obesity increased even more! As we will discuss later, when it comes to refined and processed foods, low fat is usually synonymous with high sugar. During the succeeding decades, according to government statistics, the consumption of fat has dropped about 16 percent, while the consumption of calories has remained about the same. Meanwhile, obesity has continued to climb. According to the National Center for Health Statistics, 65 percent of Americans are overweight, and 30.5 percent of us are obese.[1] Obesity, not just overweight, is now claiming 15 percent of our children.[2]

What have been the most dramatic diet and lifestyle changes in the last thirty to fifty years?

- Tremendous rise in refined sugar consumption
- Tremendous rise in low-fat foods (with, in most cases, fats being replaced with added sugars)

- Tremendous rise in carbohydrate intake as dietary fat and protein were cut
- Significant decrease in physical activity
- Tremendous rise in obesity and related illnesses
- Tremendous rise in diabetes and related illnesses
- Tremendous rise in individual dollars spent on pills, potions, and treatments

All of this and still an insignificant amount of dollars are being spent on prevention. Hello! Anybody out there? We are astonished that the government and many nutrition professionals continue to recommend high-carbohydrate, low-fat diets. As you read this book, see if you don't believe the *Sugar Busters!* lifestyle will cure many of these problems without pills or potions and their associated expenses.

By the way, we do not consider *Sugar Busters!* a low-carbohydrate lifestyle. It is simply a *correct* carbohydrate lifestyle. In our earlier fourteen-day meal plan, 40 percent of calories came from carbohydrate, and we have told people that they can probably maintain or even lose weight if they get up to 50 percent of calories from the low-glycemic-index carbohydrates. According to the chairman of the Department of Epidemiology at M. D. Anderson Hospital, the number one rated cancer research hospital in the United States,[3] the high-fiber, low-glycemic-index carbohydrates (like we recommend in our *Sugar Busters!* books) are those that are high in antioxidants and are exactly what M. D. Anderson recommends that their patients should eat.[4]

Since the *Sugar Busters!* way of eating is roughly 40 percent carbohydrates, 30 percent protein, and 30 percent fat, it is a balanced diet. According to the U.S. Department of Agriculture, a moderate-fat diet is most likely to be nutritionally adequate because it allows a healthy mix of foods from all food groups.[5] This provides a balance that does not require supplements.

Besides knowing that our digestive systems developed on a high-fiber, low-glycemic diet over the millennia, what makes the *Sugar Busters!* lifestyle tick? Controlling, which in this case means lowering, our body's insulin requirement is the key to having our body lean and healthy.

Today's sugary, highly processed foods cause a rapid rise in blood sugar, which immediately create a big demand for the hormone insulin. Insulin is required to regulate the blood sugar level in your body. It does this by signaling the cells to be receptive to the storage of fats circulating in the blood. Almost any doctor in America will tell you that insulin is known as the "fat storage hormone." Accordingly, if you consume foods that do not create this big need for insulin, you don't put the body in a fat storage mode. Neither do you subject the body to other problems caused by too much circulating insulin, as will be described further in Chapter 8.

If you enjoy eating, this is a good-news book. If you choose to eat out frequently or if your employment requires it, this is a good-news book. If you want your blood chemistry to improve while you continue to eat savory foods, this is a good-news book. If you are diabetic, this is a good-news book. If you want your children to grow up slim and healthy, this is a good-news book. In addition to all these benefits, you will feel and function better in the process. We propose a way of eating that will allow you to eat most foods in normal quantities—possibly even in larger quantities than you presently consume.

You can have three full meals a day and even appropriate snacks. If you want to eat six small meals or snacks, that's fine too. There will be only a few fruits and vegetables, plus products containing added sugars and highly processed grains (flours), that you cannot eat. These are the foods that require the secretion of large amounts of insulin to regulate your blood sugar. By simply avoiding these foods, you can get slimmer and healthier simultaneously.

There are other books that recommend a much lower percentage of carbohydrate in one's diet. Many miss one of the most important factors in successful, long-term weight loss, which is that only certain carbohydrates cause a dramatic increase in your body's need for insulin. Eliminating most carbohydrates in the diet means missing out on many of the very important vitamins, minerals, antioxidants, and other nutrients that our bodies need to function properly.

Is sugar toxic? Not inherently, but we say that refined sugar in large quantities is certainly harmful to many human bodies, particularly diabetics. And it helps make many people obese. Significant quantities of sugar are also derived in our digestive systems from carbohydrates in general (fruits, vegetables, and grains) but only certain of these sugars cause a strain on the health of our body, probably the mind, and certainly the waistline. Fructose, the sugar in fruit, normally will not hurt you, but eaten at the wrong time or in the wrong combinations, can create digestive and sometimes metabolic problems. Therefore, what we are recommending is a low-sugar, low-glycemic diet. That cannot be achieved by simply putting away your sugar canister.

The essence of the *Sugar Busters!* lifestyle, which will be covered much more thoroughly in succeeding chapters, is that the only things you cannot eat on this diet are the carbohydrates that cause an intense insulin secretion. You must virtually eliminate white potatoes, white rice, bread from highly refined flour, corn products, beets, and of course all refined sugars, such as sucrose (table sugar), corn syrup, molasses, and honey. Also, sugared soft drinks and beer are not allowed. Beyond that, the list of foods allowed on the *Sugar Busters!* lifestyle is extensive and will delight you by its length and variety.

Remember that all carbohydrates are broken down to glucose (sugar) in our body, and this raises our blood sugar level. Insulin is then secreted by the pancreas to lower our blood sugar, but too much insulin promotes the storage of fat, elevation of cholesterol levels, and possibly the deposition of plaque in our coronary arteries. Insulin also inhibits the breakdown of previously stored fat. Not fancy, but fact. The charts in Figure 1, page 18 from *Williams Textbook of Endocrinology* speak to this in a beautifully simple fashion.

By the way, some people are insulin resistant and require large quantities of insulin to regulate their blood sugar level. We have found nothing good about high average levels of insulin in the body. Insulin not only causes the body to store excess sugar as fat, but inhibits the mobilization of previously stored fat, even if one is on a rather skimpy but high-glucose-generating diet. Insulin also can stimulate the liver to make more cholesterol.

Now, you might accept the connection between insulin and overweight, but wonder about the link between insulin and cholesterol. Consider the experience of one of this book's authors.

After beginning to eat steak, lamb chops, cheese, eggs, and so on for the first time in fifteen years and seeing his cholesterol drop 21 percent and triglycerides drop by 50 percent, he told his doctor (and coauthor) that the only thing that seemed to make sense was that insulin must be causing the liver to make additional cholesterol, because the main difference his low-sugar, low-glycemic diet was causing was a lower daily average level of insulin circulating in his body. Our doctor paused about three seconds and said, "You know, you are right! When borderline diabetics get to where they cannot control their diabetes with pills, diet, and exercise, and we have to give them insulin injections, we know the first major side effect will be that their cholesterol will become elevated and as the insulin shots continue, the Type 2 diabetics also will start adding more fatty tissue."

Our doctor immediately recognized a frequently overlooked connection between insulin and cholesterol. In addition, our endocrinologist and coauthor verified that his Type 2 diabetic patients that require insulin have significantly higher total cholesterol and triglycerides than the average population.

Although we are in the twenty-first century, few appreciate the insulin-cholesterol connection. Fortunately, more and more are recognizing the link every day. Many of our friends or patients who have gone on our low-glycemic, low-sugar lifestyle have written to us that they had lowered their cholesterol by an average of 15 percent without either exercise or pills. How could they have increased their fat intake and seen their cholesterol, triglyceride, and weight levels fall? It is the effect of lower average levels of insulin in their blood.

Sound too simple? Well, it really is simple. But it's important to understand why the *Sugar Busters!* lifestyle works. Once you do, you will be confident it is not another gimmicky diet, which means you will be more likely to follow its guidelines and enjoy the maximum benefits. So please don't just jump to Chapter 9, start the diet, and then not be able to tell anybody why you lost the weight and how you got that spring back in your step. Learn how it works, and you'll better understand the benefits and enjoyment it can bring you for life—most probably a longer and healthier life.

Calories are not the only answer to weight gain or loss. Lavoisier first used the term *calorie* in the 1840s. Subsequently, in the 20th century, a caloric theory developed that explained weight gain or loss. Although this theory was later declared flawed by the authors, nutritionists ignored this correction.

We have been misled for decades by peddlers of the calorie-in-calorie-out theory, who either did not know better or had other obvious motives. The scientific data have been available in America for years, waiting for a logical researcher to come to this same conclusion. Americans alone spend $32 billion a year trying to lose weight, an additional $46 billion on medical costs directly related to problems caused by obesity, and $23 billion on time lost while away from the workplace because of the same problems. Unfortunately, for some this is an incentive to ignore a way of eating that creates no profits. So get ready—you have a lot of mis-information, misconceptions, and propaganda to overcome.

What motivates three doctors to tell you about something that will cost you only a few additional dollars each year on your grocery bill and save you the expense and time of going so often to the doctor's office? The effects of a low-glycemic diet will actually take patients away from many doctors, but doctors are in the business of saving lives. The message in this book can prolong lives and significantly improve the quality of life.

What's wrong with losing weight in other ways? Some diets are in essence partial starvation, depleting the body of essential proteins, vitamins, and minerals and making you miserable by depriving you of normal quantities of food. Of course, a whole industry is built on providing, at a price, vitamins and supplements in any quantity you might conceivably want. But did you ever taste a pill you really liked? Instead of having to swallow a pill, why not eat a plateful of savory fruits, vegetables, and meats and lose weight in the process?

What a waste of money to spend billions of dollars a year trying to lose weight. We'll show you how to replace the most notorious insulin-stimulating carbohydrates with wholesome foods that you can buy at nearly any grocery store. Watch out at the grocery store, however—manufacturers have added some form of refined sugar to most packaged products, even foods like chili, because they know that if it does not have a sweet flavor, it may not compete well with other brands.

We have harped on insulin's bad effects, but we will now describe the benefits of another of the body's secretions. Glucagon, also shown on Figure 1, page 18, is released from the pancreas into the bloodstream in significant quantities following the consumption of a protein-rich meal. Glucagon helps promote the mobilization of previously stored fat; so, as you burn food reserves for your energy requirements between meals, high levels of glucagons will help allow that energy to be derived from that spare tire around your waist. The glucagon chart also shows that, once the glucagon level is raised, it will remain elevated for quite some time so you can keep on burning that mobilized fat.

Remember, insulin inhibits the mobilization of previously stored fat. Because a high-protein meal does not stimulate significant amounts of insulin secretion, the fat mobilization inhibitor is not present, but a high level of glucagon, the fat mobilizer, *is* present.

The chart also shows that carbohydrate-rich meals actually suppress glucagon secretion. So the stored-fat mobilizer is absent, but the hormone to promote storage, insulin, is present in significant amounts. When fat gets stored, we all know where it goes!

Ready for more good news? Following the pattern of eating we recommend can greatly relieve many common stomach maladies. One of this book's authors went from Rolaids or Alka-Seltzer twice a week to none after beginning to eat steak, lamb chops, cheese, and eggs for the first time in fifteen years. The only other alteration beyond a low-sugar, low-glycemic diet that he made was the substitution of red wine for other alcoholic beverages he used to consume.

To drink or not to drink? You can find arguments both ways. But we believe, as do most American doctors, that, if you consume modest amounts of alcoholic beverages, it will help raise your HDL or "good" cholesterol, and that the alcoholic beverage that benefits you most is red wine. Populations in countries with a higher relative consumption of red wine to other spirits definitely experience a lower incidence of cardiovascular disease. Researchers believe it is primarily the polyphenols, including flavonoids, in red wine that provide the cardiovascular benefits. (See Chapter 25.)

One thing is for certain: alcohol itself has calories, so consuming it does not help you lose weight. However, with reasonably comfortable adjustments in eating habits, significant quantities of weight can be lost even if you continue to drink modest amounts of alcohol, such as red wine.

How about exercise? Exercise is a definite plus in overall body fitness and health, especially if done regularly and in moderate amounts (see Chapter 17). Nevertheless, a moderate amount of exercise will not significantly affect weight loss if you continue to eat foods that create a constant need for high levels of insulin in your bloodstream.

One of this book's authors lost twenty pounds and has kept it off for almost ten years. He's not proud that he does not take the time to exercise, but the fact is that he doesn't. So the twenty-pound weight loss did not come from exercise or a low-calorie diet. It came from a low-glycemic, low-sugar, high-fiber diet. He is not necessarily an example we want you to imitate—we definitely believe exercise is good for you. In combination with the lifestyle we recommend, it should help achieve a general improvement in body weight control and overall health.

One word of caution: If you are a marathon runner or an exercise fanatic, this diet may not be exactly right for you. High levels of exercise require foods that generate large quantities of glucose to fuel your engine. But research is showing that it is the low-glycemic-index carbs that provide the best endurance capacity.[6]

Does every person's body react to and process (metabolize) foods in exactly the same way? No, but understanding the messages in this book will help you understand not only why these differences exist, but also what you can do to positively influence your own body's reaction to various foods and combinations of foods.

Some women have found it more difficult than men to lose weight on any diet. This can be explained in part by the fact that a female's metabolic rate, on an age-adjusted basis, is usually 5 to 10 percent lower than that of a male. This makes it easier to put on weight and more difficult to lose weight. Hormonal influences present in both premenopausal and postmenopausal women also may be responsible for difficulties in losing weight. Hormone therapy, in the form of either birth control pills or estrogen and synthetic progesterone supplements, may further aggravate this problem. Chapter 16 addresses in more detail the problems some women have experienced with weight loss because of hormonal intake.

Also, please be aware that even some of the most common over-the-counter preparations can cause fluid retention, increased appetite, and other changes that can lead to weight gain. However, all individuals, especially women, should be cautions about taking or discontinuing any type of medication without prior consultation with their physicians.

How about "fat burner" supplements that are supposed to boost your metabolism even in the absence of exercise? According to the *Tufts University*

*Health and Nutrition Letter* of May 2002, almost all contain ephedra, which can increase your metabolism, but can also cause irregular heartbeat, high blood pressure, chest pain, and even stroke, heart attack, seizures, and death. Ephedra is marketed as a dietary supplement rather than a drug, and supplements are not regulated, unlike prescription drugs, so buyer beware.

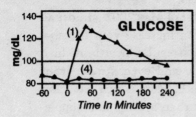

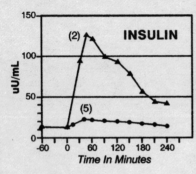

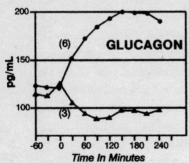

▲ **High-carbohydrate meal**
● **High-protein meal**

## Figure 1.

Following a high-carbohydrate meal, glucose levels rise rapidly (1), stimulating the release of insulin (2), which promotes utilization of glucose but also signals the body to store fat and prevent the mobilization of previously stored fat. Glucagon secretion is suppressed by the high glucose level (3). A high-protein meal, however, causes only an imperceptible rise in blood glucose (4) and, consequently, a very small rise in insulin (5), but a significant increase in the glucagon level (6). Glucagon promotes the mobilization of previously stored fat.

Source: Modified from Wilson and Foster (1992).

## 2 | The Glycemic Index

The glycemic index (GI) is a measure of how much a specific amount of ingested carbohydrate (usually 50 grams) will cause a person's blood sugar to rise and remain elevated over time, relative to the effect on blood sugar of the same amount of pure glucose (which is assigned a GI of 100). To determine a food's glycemic index, the food and glucose are consumed on separate days, blood samples are taken under supervised conditions, and the results are measured in a laboratory. The measurements are precise and scientifically straightforward. To allow for metabolic variation within a given individual, the testing is repeated at least once on different days. To allow for the natural variation in metabolic reaction between individuals, the glycemic index testing is usually done on at least twelve individuals, and then averaged to come up with the final number.

Might the final number vary somewhat for different groups of twelve people? It probably would, slightly. Might the ethnic background and historical dietary environment of different people cause a variation? It probably would. In the future, as more GI responses are measured on many more people, the GIs that fit your group will become more accurate. All that said, the relative GIs as published today are still good indicators of how a given amount of a specific food will affect your blood sugar and also of the amount of insulin required to bring your blood sugar back to normal.

One factor that causes variation in GI results is that different variants of the same type of fruit, grain, or vegetable can cause, in some instances, fairly large differences in the glycemic reaction. For instance, sweet corn from New Zealand has been measured to have a GI of 48, while sweet corn from an American grocery store has been measured to have a GI of 60. Similarly, an orange bought in Denmark has a GI of 31, while an orange bought in Canada measures 51.[1] Variation can also occur in the GI measurement of individual foods of the same type grown within the continental United States. Also, the ripeness of fruit can cause variation. Ripe bananas have a higher GI than less ripe, greenish bananas.

We feel that a very important determinant of the glycemic index is the particle size and form in which a carboydrate comes packaged by nature. Cracked grains produce a lower glycemic index than coarse flour, which in turn produces a lower glycemic index than finely milled flour (Figure 2, page 21). The lowest glycemic indexes are associated with the whole grains.[2] It is no surprise that

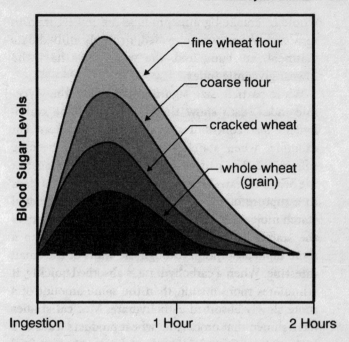

*The larger the particle size, the lower the glycemic index*

**Figure 2.**

## Effects of processing grain

whole or cracked grains produce the lowest insulin response. When whole, rolled, or finely milled oats (oatmeal) are compared, the whole oats have the lowest glycemic index.

While particle size significantly affects the glycemic index, data show that the form of the carbohydrate also contributes to glycemic differences. For example, when starches are cooked, they become gelatinized. The particles or granules swell because of the heat and water absorbed during cooking. This leads to a rupture of the granule, exposing the individual starch molecules, thus increasing the susceptibility of the starch to enzymatic digestion. This leads to a more rapid absorption through the walls of the small intestine. When a carbohydrate is absorbed quickly, it stimulates more insulin than the same amount of a more slowly absorbed carbohydrate. Medical studies have shown that processing wheat products leads to a higher glycemic index for these foods. Modern food processing may include puffing, thermal extrusion, intense mechanical treatments, and canning, all of which alter the foods to a considerable degree. Generally, products with the least degree of processing have the lowest glycemic index. Therefore, the more processing a carbohydrate such as rice, corn, or wheat has been subjected to, the higher its glycemic index.

An interesting and useful point is that the addition of vinegar or even lemon or lime juice has been reported to lower the glycemic effect of a meal.

People who have access to a glucose monitor can

determine their approximate glycemic reaction to a specific food by testing themselves after fasting and then testing themselves after eating the food.

Bottom line? We believe that choosing foods based on their relative GIs is a very valuable way to help select the foods that will help you control your weight and also provide you with the vitamins, minerals, antioxidants, and other nutrients that you need for optimum health.

We are not alone in this view. Dr. David S. Ludwig of Harvard, director of the obesity program at Children's Hospital in Boston maintains that the GI has value in helping people choose a healthful diet. He cautions, however, as we do, that you also need to take into account how much of a particular food you eat.[3] Dr. Susan Roberts, professor of nutrition at Tufts University, says, "I am personally convinced that low-GI diets help people lose weight," and GI researcher Dr. Christine L. Pelkman of Pennsylvania State University says, "We're learning that the type of carbs you eat really makes a difference in your health" and that "the glycemic index helps you choose the best carbs for you."[4]

Dr. Christiane Northrup, author of an excellent book titled *The Wisdom of Menopause*, writes favorably about the application of the glycemic index for choosing the proper foods. In her book she lists *Sugar Busters!* as one of the few books on diet or lifestyle that she recommends you read and follow for a healthy diet.

We consume large quantities of some carbohydrates in an average serving size and small quantities of other carbohydrates. We alluded to the powerful blood sugar raising impact of eating a baked white potato in our earlier book. An average-size baked white potato weighs around 8 ounces. Since a white potato is approximately 35 percent carbohydrate, that calculates to about 80 grams of carbohydrate with a very high GI of 95. If you want to compare the potato's blood-sugar-stimulating effect relative to table sugar, which has a GI of 65,[5] you find that it would take 118 grams of sugar to have the same impact as the potato. That is 29½ teaspoons of sugar! (A 6-ounce potato calculates to 22 teaspoons and a 10-ounce potato to 37 teaspoons of sugar.) If you still decide to eat a white potato, please eat the skin, which contains nearly all the potato's fiber and many of its nutrients. For an excellent substitution for a white potato, a 1-cup serving of cooked lentils, with a GI of only 28, results in an impact of only 4⅓ teaspoons of table sugar. The glycemic response for most dried beans would be similar, although somewhat higher.

Do not be afraid of getting some sugar through your carbohydrates, however. That is where you get your energy. The problem simply lies in the fact that a serving of a high-glycemic-index food can give you so much sugar and potential energy that a lot can be left over to turn to fat.

By the way, the critics were right! A carrot, albeit with a high GI, is 93 percent water and only 7 percent carbohydrate so a carrot eaten in normal quantities will not give you a large blood-sugar stimulating reaction despite its high GI. So, enjoy the nutritive benefits of modest portions of carrots from time to time.

Harvard has proposed measuring foods by their glycemic load (GL). It is measured simply by multiplying the grams of carbohydrates in an average-size serving of a given food times the GI of that same food.[6] It is reasonable, logical, and we support it as another useful tool in the glycemic approach to choosing the right carbohydrates to eat. Sometime in the future, we predict, GIs and GLs for overall meals will be widely available for a broad range of foods and can further help you in planning and selecting your meals.

One more time, regarding the consumption of so much refined table sugar: There are no vitamins, minerals, trace elements, or fiber in table sugar, only empty calories.

## Figure 3.
## Glycemic Index

(Compiled from multiple glycemic studies. Measurements on American grain products, fruits, and vegetables are used if available. The numbers are rounded since results vary somewhat from individual to individual or group to group.

### Grains, Breads, and Cereals

It is very difficult to find breakfast cereals that are processed without the addition of one or more sugars. Some cereal flakes are even sugar-coated. We recommend whole-grain breads that have the intact or cracked kernel as much as possible. The higher the percentage (50 perecnt or more), the better.

Another problem is found in breads that contain enriched flour. This means the grain initially has been so highly processed that even the vitamins and minerals have been stripped out and must be replaced (enriched). Read the labels closely and go with those that have very little or no added sugar, the highest fiber or bran content, and the least processing of the grains. Also avoid corn-based cereals.

Of the pastas, stone-ground whole-grain pasta would be the best. Next-best would be a coarse, stone-ground whole-wheat pasta.

| **HIGH** | | | |
|---|---|---|---|
| White bread | 75–95 | Corn | 75 |
| French bread | 75 | Corn chips | 75 |
| Cornflakes | 90 | Graham crackers | 75 |
| Instant rice | 90 | Regular crackers | 75 |
| Rice cakes | 80–90 | Bagel, white flour | 75 |
| Pretzels, white flour | 80 | Total cereal | 75 |
| Rice Krispies | 80 | Cheerios | 75 |

| | | | |
|---|---|---|---|
| Puffed wheat | 75 | Wild rice | 55 |
| Grape Nuts | 75 | Brown rice | 55 |
| English muffin | 75 | Oatmeal | 55 |
| Croissant | 70 | Muesli, no sugar added | 55 |
| White rice | 70 | Whole-grain | |
| Taco shells | 70 | pumpernickel | 50 |
| Cream of Wheat | 70 | Cracked-wheat | |
| Shredded wheat | 70 | bulgur bread | 50 |
| Special K | 70 | High % cracked-wheat | |
| Melba toast | 70 | bread | 50 |
| Millet | 70 | Whole rice | 50 |
| Whole-wheat crackers | 65 | Oat and bran bread | 50 |
| | | Sponge cake | 45 |
| Nutri-grain cereal | 65 | Pita bread, stone-ground | |
| Stoned Wheat Thins | 65 | whole-wheat | 45 |
| Regular pasta | 65 | Wheat grain | 45 |
| Raisin bran | 60 | Barley grain | 45 |
| Couscous | 60 | Whole-grain pasta | 45 |
| Corn meal | 70 | All Bran, no sugar added | 45 |
| Basmati rice | 60 | Whole-grain spaghetti | 40 |
| Spaghetti, white flour | 60 | | |
| | | **LOW** | |
| **MODERATE** | | Rye grain | 35 |
| Pita bread, regular | 55 | | |
| Rye bread, sourdough | 55 | | |

## Vegetables

Most vegetables are very good in providing much of the natural carbohydrates we definitely should include in our daily diets. A few, however, do stimulate excessive insulin secretion and should be avoided. For a more complete listing of the acceptable vegetables, please refer to Figure 9 (pages 93–94).

| HIGH | | LOW | |
|---|---|---|---|
| Baked potato | 95 | Dried beans | 30–40 |
| Mashed potato | 95 | Pinto beans | 40 |
| Parsnips | 95 | Green beans | 40 |
| Carrots | 85* | Chickpeas | 35 |
| French fries | 80 | Lima beans | 30 |
| Beets | 75 | Black beans | 30 |
| Sweet corn | 60 | Butter beans | 30 |
| | | Kidney beans | 30 |
| **MODERATE** | | Lentils | 30 |
| Sweet potatoes | 55 | Soybeans | 15 |
| Yams | 50 | Green vegetables | |
| Green peas | 45 | (Fig. 9, 93–94) | 0–15 |
| Black-eyed peas | 40 | | |

* The carbs in carrots have a high glycemic index, but only about 7% of a carrot by weight is carbohydrate, so moderate amounts of carrots are okay.

## Fruits

Fruits are a great source of sugar because they generally have a moderate to low insulin-stimulating effect and also provide vitamins necessary to good health. As explained, however, fruits are handled best by our digestive system if consumed alone. While not individually listed, fruit juices generally have a modestly higher glycemic index than the whole fruit itself.

| HIGH | | | |
|---|---|---|---|
| Watermelon | 70 | Banana, green | 45 |
| Pineapple | 65 | Peaches | 40 |
| Raisins | 65 | Plums | 40 |
| Bananas, ripe | 60 | Apples | 40 |
| | | Oranges | 40 |
| MODERATE | | Apple juice | 40 |
| Orange juice, from | | | |
| concentrate | 55 | LOW | |
| Mango | 50 | Apricots, dried | 30 |
| Kiwi | 50 | Grapefruit | 25 |
| Grapes | 50 | Cherries | 25 |
| Plantains | 45 | Tomatoes | 15 |
| Pears | 45 | Apricots, fresh | 10 |
| Orange juice, fresh | 45 | | |

## Dairy Products

Dairy products also provide many of the vitamins necessary to good health. Furthermore, except for dairy products with added sugar, they all possess a moderate to low insulin-stimulating effect. But please don't overdo the amount of saturated fat consumed through dairy products.

| HIGH | | | |
|---|---|---|---|
| Ice cream, premium | 60 | Milk, whole | >30 |
| | | Milk, skim | <30 |
| **MODERATE** | | Yogurt, plain, no sugar | 15 |
| Yogurt, with added fruit | 35 | | |

## Miscellaneous

| HIGH | | LOW | |
|---|---|---|---|
| Maltose (as in beer) | 105 | Nuts | 15–30 |
| Glucose | 100 | Peanuts | 15 |
| Honey | 65 | | |
| Refined sugar | 65 | | |
| Popcorn | 55 | | |

Recently, Harvard Medical School's *Harvard Heart Letter* (December 2002, page 4) reported that the World Health Organization and the National Institute of Medicine favor use of the glycemic index in choosing healthy foods. *Sugar Busters!* first made that recommendation in 1995!

# 3 | A Brief History of Refined Sugar

In all the eons over which our digestive systems were evolving, the world simply did not have refined sugar or refined, high-glycemic carbohydrates—yet our ancestors thrived, even though they lived in harsh physical conditions. In some places a little honey or sugar cane might have been available occasionally, but most of the world's inhabitants had no refined sugar at all—not in all those hundreds of thousands of years.

Early on, our ancestors did not even have the luxury of being able to eat a combination of foods. They ate like all animals eat today (unless we force our pets to eat otherwise)—only one thing at a time, and that was in a completely unrefined form. They did not eat the kind of carbohydrates that would require large amounts of insulin secretion. The staples of our diet today—white bread, white rice, white potatoes, refined flours, refined sugars, hybridized fruits and vegetables, and soft drinks—were not available. For hundreds of millennia, our ancestors ate only a low-glycemic diet. Back then, the pancreas was probably not called upon to secrete as much insulin in one day of an entire lifetime as it is called upon to secrete nearly every day of our modern post-infant lifetime!

For a visual example of how we have come in just the last fifteen centuries from zero refined sugar intake to today's average daily consumption of refined sugar alone, see Figure 4 (page 33). Think of how much more glucose (sugar) is generated with the carbohydrate and starch combinations of our "balanced American diet," like a baked white potato, that does not ever get picked up in the comparative statistics!

We have had refined sugar only for a mere blink of time in humans' digestive evolution. Think about it—refined sugar and refined flour are "new" foods. Is it any wonder that the incidence of diabetes and impaired glucose tolerance continues to get higher and higher? Maybe we eat too much sugar and simply wear out or exhaust our pancreas glands, which surely did not evolve to produce the quantities of insulin a typical modern diet demands.

Refined sugar did not exist anywhere in the world until around A.D. 500. The old holy books of the world's leading religions do not even mention sugar. Honey, yes; sugar, no. The early writers and historians did not have a word for it. If they had, they surely would have mentioned it prominently, as every society introduced to refined sugar has been immediately hooked on its delights and, unfortu-

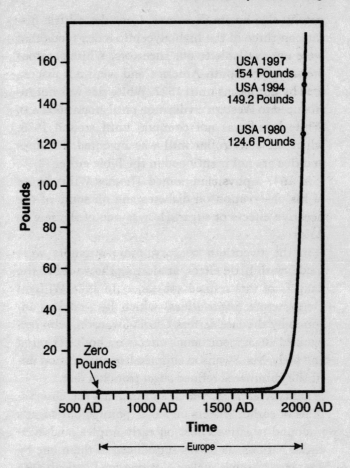

**Figure 4.**

**Total refined sugar consumption per person per year.**

Source: U.S. Department of Agriculture.

nately, also on its ill effects. Consider a little history on three of the high-glycemic-index foods that were not available to our ancestors. White potatoes are native to South America and were not discovered by Europeans until 1537. White rice was not introduced to Western civilization until around 600 A.D. White bread was not common until around 1875, when the steel roller mill was invented. Potatoes and rice are not mentioned in the Bible either.

In 1647 a physician named Thomas Willis wrote of his observation on diabetes and on some of the negative effects of sugar. He was one of the few to do so.

In the twentieth century, more attempts were made, with little effect, at alerting the world to the dangers of this refined substance. In 1976 William Dufty wrote *Sugar Blues*, which he said was inspired by the late actress Gloria Swanson, who recognized sugar's poisonous effects on both her mind and body. Ms. Swanson suffered from depression until she eliminated refined sugar from her diet.

Dufty's research, which summarized the observations of earlier writers on sugar, pointed out sugar's profound negative effect on early armies, and even entire nations, as it was introduced to them one by one. His research makes a strong (and logical) case that the incidence of diabetes and other diseases grew significantly as refined sugar consumption increased.

Why have the early physicians' and anti-sugar

crusaders' insights and observations never caught on? The refined-sugar lobby has been very powerful for a couple of centuries. The economic stakes in the sugar trade between nations were extremely high. Slavery even flourished because of it. Pro-sugar lobbying by sugar growers, soft-drink manufacturers, and the packaged-food industry has been very effective in influencing our government. What politician wants to tell his or her constituents that they should no longer eat sugar?

Is it wrong to lobby for one's own product? No, but it is wrong to minimize the very serious side effects of too much refined-sugar consumption, such as causing a higher incidence of diabetes, a very serious disease with severe consequences for many of our organs.

The main problem with society's ignorance of sugar's evil effects probably lies in our tendency to ignore what we do not want to hear. Information about the health problems sugar can cause has been out there, but people simply did not want to hear the message. Like alcoholics hooked on alcohol, our society is hooked on sugar. People say, "Just don't tell me that sugar is bad, too!"

Yet when we initially self-published our book, it took only a little over two years to see more than 200,000 copies sold and for it to build up a legion of successful followers. As the book was not advertised, the buzz must have come by word of mouth. Following the success of that early book and prior to the sale of this current book, the professionally published hardcover version of *Sugar Busters! Cut Sugar to Trim Fat* leapt to the number-one spot on the *New York Times* bestseller list, remained there for months, and sold well in excess of two million copies. People simply needed a simple, straightforward explanation of how consumption of sugar and other high-glycemic-index carbohydrates was really going to make them fat (and unhealthy).

There is some interesting information on average life span that might surprise you. The statistic that men's life expectancy has increased by 50 percent in the last century is accurate, but is misleading in that it is nearly all due to a tremendous decrease in infant and early childhood mortality. Middle-aged American men only live a couple of years longer on average than they did in 1900, despite the availability of flu shots, penicillin for pneumonia, antibiotics, early detection technology, transplant capability, and multiple life-support systems (all of which, admittedly, can make a difference in individual cases, but we are concerned with population-wide statistics here).

We also have refrigeration and improved packaging technology, which allow us to eat a wide variety of food all year. And you cannot go into any food store or drugstore without finding shelves and shelves of vitamins, minerals, and other supplements.

Why doesn't all this preventive medicine, year-round availability of a balanced diet, and life-support technology result in more than a two-year extension of an average middle-aged man's life?

We believe the main culprit is the major change to refined foods, including refined sugar. This has done to our entire population exactly what it did to royalty over the last few centuries. The privileged could afford white bread and lots of sugar, which rapidly took a toll by making them fat and giving them gout and diabetes. Just because we have everything in the world to eat doesn't mean we really eat better or even as well as most of our forefathers who ate in the fashion for which their digestive systems were designed. In fact, we believe that a middle-aged man's general quality of life despite the medical wonders, has diminished. The miraculous medical advances have been offset by the tremendous rise in sugar intake, as shown in Figure 4 (page 33) and the consumption of other high-glycemic, low-fiber foods.

When you see the increase in disease caused by our huge consumption of refined sugar and certain other carbohydrates, it is quite logical to add refined sugar to the priority list of things that are or may be hazardous to your health. Too much sugar just may be the number-one culprit in lowering quality of life and causing premature death. There certainly is enough evidence to bring us to that conclusion.

If the sugar-causes-disease message has not caught on yet, why do we think another book about it is worth the effort? Excess insulin is causing problems that can kill people prematurely, and even those who survive to an older age often have a greatly reduced quality of life. The importance of insulin was ignored in the vast majority of nutritional and dietetic literature until just very recently. The "insulin connection" needs to be better understood and must be told over and over until it is appreciated.

You can benefit from a low-sugar diet. One of the good old clichés is very applicable here: "Today is the first day of the rest of your life." Think about it.

Finally, the basic principles outlined in *Sugar Busters!* have been field-tested by the human digestive system throughout the eons. The *Sugar Busters!* lifestyle is unlike recent diet and supplement programs that are long on promise but short on proof. These new claims are all too often proven to be false or ineffective after a few years of research. Worse yet, some of these diet plans and pills turn out to be dangerous to our health. But every time a new gimmick gets widely publicized, someone makes a ton of money from the sales attached to it. In contrast, following the principles of the *Sugar Busters!* lifestyle costs essentially nothing.

# 4 | Calculating Fatness and Obesity

How do you know whether you or your children are of normal body weight or are fat or obese? You cannot always tell simply by your appearance, or your children's, or by comparison with others, because the weights of adults and children have increased dramatically over the past few decades, and as populations become heavier, the perception of what is normal weight changes. The body mass index (BMI) is a standardized tool to determine the amount of body fat both in adults and children.

The body mass index is a calculation of a person's weight relative to height. The BMI can be calculated by dividing weight in pounds by height in inches, dividing that result by height in inches again, and finally multiply that result by 703. For example, if your weight is 140 pounds and your height is 5 feet (60 inches), the calculation would be as follows: $140 \div 60 = 2.33$, then $2.33 \div 60 = .0388$, and $.0388 \times 703 = 27.2764$. Rounding down, that produces a BMI of 27.

In adults, since height is fixed, the BMI changes

only with weight. A BMI equal to or greater than 25 in adults indicates overweight. A BMI equal to or greater than 30 indicates obesity. Those potential complications of overweight and obesity can be found in Chapter 6.

For children, go ahead and calculate their BMI as you did for yourself. However, since the weights and heights of children change with age, the BMI changes until growth is complete. The Centers for Disease Control have gathered data on children relative to height, weight, and age to calculate their BMI percentiles. For male and female children age 2 to 20, their intersection of their age and BMI can be found in Figures 5 and 6, pages 42 and 43. A child whose BMI versus age plots at or above the 85th percentile (that is, he or she weighs more than 85 percent of children of the same age, height, and sex) is considered to be overweight. Any child whose BMI is at or above the 95th percentile is considered to be obese, and this obesity is very likely to persist into adulthood. Approximately 25 percent of children in the United States are overweight or obese. (Note that the BMI charts may not work for a small number of children—for instance, some athletic, muscular children may have a normal amount of body fat yet have a high BMI, and children who are very inactive may have a normal BMI but an unhealthy amount of body fat. In spite of these limitations, the BMI is considered to be extremely useful in identifying weight problems in most children. Consult your child's pediatrician if you have any concerns.)

You can also use the calculators at the Centers for Disease Control Web site to calculate your BMI. These are found on the Internet at www.cdc.gov/nccdphp/dnpa/bmil/calc-bmi.htm and www.cdc.gov/nccdphp/dnpa/bmi/bmi-for-age.htm.

BMI can be a useful tool for determining whether you are at risk for the complications of overweight and obesity. *The Sugar Busters!* way of eating will help you and your children achieve and maintain a normal, healthy weight.

The medical literature is now full of studies that indicate the following health problems are more prevalent in significantly overweight and obese people.

| | |
|---|---|
| Type I diabetes | Eating disorders |
| CV disease, strokes | Indigestion |
| High blood pressure | Migraine headaches |
| Elevated cholesterol | Polycystic ovaries |
| Elevated triglycerides | Stress |
| Asthma | Certain cancers |
| Sleep apnea | Low self-esteem |
| Incontinence | Depression |
| | Suicide |

**Figure 5.**

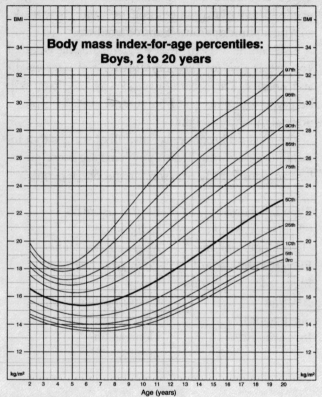

Body mass index-for-age percentiles:
Boys, 2 to 20 years

SOURCE: Developed by the National Center for Health Statistics in collaboration with
the National Center for Chronic Disease Prevention and Health Promotion (2000).

**Figure 6.**

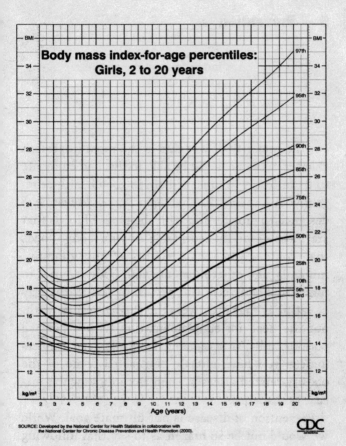

Body mass index-for-age percentiles: Girls, 2 to 20 years

SOURCE: Developed by the National Center for Health Statistics in collaboration with the National Center for Chronic Disease Prevention and Health Promotion (2000).

# 5 | Prevention

For the majority of you this is the most important chapter in the book. To be able to live and enjoy life to its fullest, you must remain in good health or regain your lost health. The *Sugar Busters!* lifestyle is designed to provide you with the types of foods that are most naturally acceptable to your body—foods that contain generous amounts of the vitamins, minerals, and other nutrients your body requires to function effectively. The best thing about this way of eating is that it delivers the desired results without the need for supplementation with expensive potions, pills, or assistance from personal trainers (unless you have already contracted some of the obesity-related diseases, such as cardiovascular disease or diabetes).

Prevention of disease is our ultimate goal. While we would not be so brazen as to say that following the *Sugar Busters!* lifestyle will prevent all the problems a body might develop, we are simply saying it is loaded with the good foods that have successfully nurtured our forebears through the eons when no medical help existed.

To get started, let's talk about prevention of diabetes. Suppose a laboratory blood test could tell you that sometime in the future your chance of developing Type 2 diabetes is very high. There is no doubt that FACING THE PROSPECT OF HAVING A HEART ATTACK, STROKE, LOSS OF VISION, OR AMPUTATION IS VERY FRIGHTENING. But there is hope to prevent this deadly disease. A blood test can help determine whether most people are already pre-diabetic. If anything you read in this chapter or in Chapter 13 makes you think you may have pre-diabetes or diabetes, go have your blood tested immediately.

Recent scientific publications have revealed the causes and risk factors leading to the development of Type 2 diabetes. A diet that is loaded with high-glycemic carbohydrates can not only cause pancreatic exhaustion by repeated demands on the pancreas to release large amounts of insulin but such a diet also promotes the condition of insulin resistance. Insulin resistance often precedes the development of Type 2 diabetes. A person who has insulin resistance requires higher levels of insulin to maintain a normal blood sugar.

The United States in the late 20th and early 21th century, with its high-glycemic, Western diet, has become an ideal laboratory or culture medium for producing diabetics. Our baby boomers that have grown up on this diet are reaching the ages (late 50's and early 60's) when most persons are first diagnosed with diabetes. More than ever, our overweight children are reaching adulthood overweight and with a higher risk for the development of Type 2 diabetes as compared to their parents. The population within many ethnic groups also is increasing rapidly and many are at unusually high risk for developing the disease. Later in this chapter we will give advice on how to prevent the development of Type 2 diabetes.

Well over 90 percent of the dollars spent by our government on health care are spent on treatment of illnesses. Little is spent on advising people how to not get sick in the first place. Other than our government's food pyramid (which was heavily influenced by lobbying from many powerful food manufacturers and which clearly did not work) or the "don't eat fat or junk food" approach, the general population has had to rely on what manufacturers and the pill and potion pushers have plied us with in copious amounts of advertising.

Much of this advertising, whether in the media or printed on the packaging, has been subjected to minimal government scrutiny. Formal studies have not been done to prove or disprove most of the claims made by the peddlers of the information. We have all heard of the problems caused by inadequate long-term testing of many products that were championed as miracles, only to later be the subject of lawsuits because of the harm they caused. Why not keep yourself out of harm's way by simply eating a good variety of the more natural foods that the human body has functioned well on for centuries and centuries?

The best way to obtain nutrients is through natural fruits, vegetables, meats, grains, nuts, dairy, and other foods instead of through pills or potions. Think of the new things now being found to be important to our health that were not recognized just a few short years ago, such as homocysteine, lysine, and lycopene. Most doctors, nutritionists, and scientists agree that we will continue to find other elements in our foods that may be playing important roles in our overall health. Two things are for certain: if a nutrient is not currently recognized, you will not find it in a pill, but if you are eating a good variety of healthful foods, your body will extract those nutrients to be used for your benefit, just as it has over the eons.

If you do not exercise, and we strongly recommend that you do, you can at least get all of the benefits of eating a healthy diet. Do not say to yourself, "Well, I won't exercise, so I guess I'll just give up and get fat." Many, many people have lost or stabilized their weight just by eating the proper foods.

Following are two examples of studies that will get you to thinking about prevention. A cover story in *Newsweek* of September 4, 2000, by Jerry Adler and Claudia Kalb, did a good job of summarizing recent statistics concerning diabetes: "Eighty-five percent of all diabetes sufferers are overweight or obese. A study by the Centers for Disease Control and Prevention found that diagnosed cases of diabetes increased by a third between 1990 and 1998. The most alarming statistic in the CDC study was that the incidence of diabetes increased 40 percent over the eight years and for people in their 30's, it went up nearly 70 percent. Further, in 1991 only seven states had obesity rates over 15 percent, while by 1998, 45 states had rates of obesity above 15 percent. States with diabetes rates over six percent jumped from nine states to 22 states from 1991 to 1998."

A study of more than one million people sponsored by the American Cancer Society found that simply being overweight can cause a higher incidence of cancer and heart disease and can cut your life short.[1] "It [the study] settles once and for all any lingering questions about whether weight alone increases the risk of death and disease," said Dr. Jo Ann Manson, a Harvard University endocrinologist and preventative-health specialist.[2]

The *Newsweek* article and the American Cancer Society study did a real service by further alerting people to the epidemic of obesity and diabetes and the problems they cause. We agree that obesity and the incidence of diabetes are closely related. The primary goal of *Sugar Busters!* is to help people of all ages not to get overweight or obese in the first place. For those who have already contracted diabetes or are obese and at high risk, the *Sugar Busters!* lifestyle of consuming low-glycemic, high-fiber carbohydrates is the best preventative program we can recommend.

Let's examine some of the types of problems that we believe frequently can be avoided by simply changing the way you eat.

*Diabetes:* Diabetes is much more prevalent in overweight or obese people. The Harvard Nurses Health Study found that people who ate low-glycemic-index, high-fiber carbohydrates, like those recommended in *Sugar Busters!*, had a 250 percent less risk of contracting diabetes. To ignore the results of this huge, long-term study, you really are playing with fire.

To prevent Type 2 diabetes, follow the *Sugar Busters!* eating plan, lose enough of your body weight to get your body mass index below 25, eat fewer trans fats and saturated fats, stop smoking, eat more whole grains and fiber, and exercise several days a week. A recent study using data from the Health Professionals Follow-up Study that began in 1986 concluded that "in men, a diet high in whole grains is associated with a lower risk of Type 2 diabetes. Efforts should be made to replace refined-grain with whole-grain foods."[3] You will move from a high-risk group to a low-risk group and, hopefully, never develop Type 2 diabetes. See Chapter 13 for further discussion.

*Cardiovascular disease:* Dr. Gerald Berenson, who has led the world-renowned Bogalusa Heart Study for over thirty years, found that the earliest reliable indicator of future cardiovascular disease was observing an increase in blood serum levels of insulin. A low-glycemic diet, like that recommended in *Sugar Busters!*, never causes much of a rise in insulin levels in the first place.

*Hypoglycemia (low blood sugar):* The authors have been contacted over and over by people who have cured their problem with low blood sugar by switching to the *Sugar Busters!* lifestyle. See Chapter 14 for further discussion.

*Stroke:* The bioflavonoids and some other natural antioxidants found in many low- and moderate-glycemic carbohydrates help make the platelets in the blood less adhesive and less prone to clotting, which is the major cause of stroke.

*Kidney disease:* Diabetics have a much higher incidence of renal (kidney) disease than nondiabetics.[4]

*Poor circulation:* Again, this is a problem much more common in people with diabetes, and it can lead to amputation.

*Depression:* Blood sugar swings can certainly aggravate, if not cause, depression in some people. See *Sugar Blues* by Michael Duffy.

*Elevated triglycerides and cholesterol:* Many,

many *Sugar Busters!* followers have experienced a drop in both triglyceride and cholesterol levels once they started eating a low-glycemic regimen that lowered their daily need for as much insulin.

The following is an illustration of what a good diet can achieve for someone with a serious blood sugar and cholesterol problem. Jerry Jordan, from Columbus, Ohio, is immediate past chairman of the national Independent Producers Association of America, and this is his story.

Jerry told one of our authors in 1999 that he was having an extended problem with his triglycerides which were extremely high (1,410!) and that he had become allergic to the various medications, including Lipitor, that were being administered by his doctor. His cholesterol was also high (240), he was somewhat overweight, and he was beginning to wonder just how long he would live. After being given a copy of *Sugar Busters! Cut Sugar to Trim Fat* by one of our authors, Jerry decided to change his way of eating and found that, without medication, he could reduce his blood fats and cholesterol dramatically. Within a few months, Jerry's triglyceride levels had dropped from 1,410 to 320, his cholesterol was down from 240 to 186, and although weight loss was not his original goal, he did lose 28 pounds! Three years later, except for occasional temporary rises, Jerry's triglycerides are still averaging only 250, his cholesterol is still in the 180s, and he has successfully retained his weight loss. He credits the *Sugar Busters!* lifestyle with causing a dramatic turn around in his blood chemistries.

Just think of all the complications that probably have been prevented by Jerry simply eating in a way that dramatically lowered his blood fats and cholesterol.

*Osteoporosis:* A recent study by researchers at Creighton University of ninety-six women age sixty-five and older found that those who drank more than three cups of coffee containing caffeine had more osteoporotic problems than the women who drank three cups or less. In a three-year period, those who drank over three cups per day lost significantly more spinal bone and, in fact, more bone throughout their body.[5]

*Cancer:* Being overweight not only increases the risk of cancer but decreases the chance of survival after getting cancer.[6]

All of the above health problems can and usually do cause a greatly diminished quality of life or even premature death. If preventing them were very painful, like sticking a long needle in the stomach every day, one might say, "Well, the heck with prevention!" But switching to the *Sugar Busters!* lifestyle and having to avoid only a handful of foods clearly is not painful. So get on with the prevention!

## 6 | The Epidemic of Childhood Obesity (and What to do About It)

Listen up, mothers, fathers, grandparents, and friends. The U.S. Surgeon General in 1998 declared childhood obesity a national epidemic. Your young ones are getting fat and sick. Obesity in children has doubled in the last decade. Statistically, fat children become fat adults. Sixty percent of fat children have health problems directly related to being fat. The more a child (or adult) is overweight, the greater the occurrence of related health problems. Even those overweight or obese children who appear to be healthy today are laying the groundwork for an adulthood that is likely to have a greatly diminished quality of life.

Type 2 diabetes, which used to be seen almost exclusively in adults (and which was also called "adult-onset diabetes" for just that reason), has tripled in children in the last decade. Diabetes is a devastating disease for children as well as adults. While genetics plays a part in one's susceptibility to contracting diabetes, genetics alone cannot account for this sudden surge in the incidence of Type 2 diabetes in our children. On the other hand, the increase in childhood diabetes is following the sudden surge in childhood obesity. See Chapter 13 for a discussion of the problems diabetes causes in adults.

The following other diseases or problems are more common in overweight and obese children:

- Heart attacks
- High blood pressure
- Elevated cholesterol
- Elevated triglycerides
- Asthma
- Orthopedic problems
- Sleep apnea
- Eating disorders
- Low self-esteem
- Depression
- Suicide

Also, pathology reports show that 25 percent of nineteen-year-olds nationwide show early symptoms of hardening of the arteries (arteriosclerosis). Poor diet and elevated insulin levels are thought by many to be the prime contributors to these shocking statistics.

While you may think we are trying to scare you to death with the above, we are merely reporting the facts. We think you might see why we have recently written a book on children's problems with obesity, *Sugar Busters! for Kids*. The new book contains specific meal plans for children, new research information, charts and formulas to determine your child's body mass index (BMI), and illustrated rhymes to help your child learn the principles of good eating habits, and it emphasizes the harm done by the terrible trio of sodas, french fries, and candy.

What can you do about your children's eating habits? At a very early age, you can do almost everything, but as they grow older, you will have less and less influence. However, less does not mean none. The main thing to do is to be a role model for them—tell them what to do and then do it yourself. Beyond that, keep the wrong things out of your kitchen and pantry. The things that are bad for them are the same things we say to avoid in this book.

For a real short list of foods to avoid, follow this advice. Eliminate sugar-sweetened soft drinks, french fries, white potatoes, white rice, white bread, corn, candy, and added sugars. Despite what the purists commonly claim, government studies continue to find no significant problems for humans from consumption of either aspartame- or saccharine-based sweeteners. If you prefer natural sweeteners, use stevia or fructose.

We have covered the dietary consequences of a poor diet relative to obese and fat children. Exercise also plays a key role. Children simply are not getting enough exercise at home or at school. You can and should try to change that at home and at school. In 2001, the Surgeon General reported that only 25 percent of high school students participated in daily physical education.[1] Some schools in America no longer even offer recess or organized physical activities. Set limits on TV viewing and other sedentary activities when they come home.

In a study conducted at the University of Miami School of Medicine, researchers found that adolescents who exercised regularly have higher grades and better relationships with their parents than do their less active peers. The active children also have a lower incidence of depression and are less likely to use drugs.[2]

Children are easy targets for shrewd marketers. When you see them being urged to eat something unhealthy, point it out to them. This will eventually teach them to be wary of media advertising and help them be more discerning throughout life. Dr. Marion Nestle, chairman of the Department of Nutrition at New York University and author of *Food Politics*, points out that only 20 percent of the food dollar goes to the farmer, while 80 percent goes to advertising.

Most of all, be a good role model for your children and their friends. Your sphere of influence might be wider than you think. Stress healthy eating instead of dieting (particularly crash dieting). Remember that the *Sugar Busters!* eating plan will satisfy their appetite. A study of low-glycemic diets versus a reduced-fat diet with an equal amount of calories on 107 obese but otherwise healthy children by Dr. David S. Ludwig, director of the obesity program at Children's Hospital in Boston, found that body mass index (BMI) decreased more in the low-glycemic diet (like that recommended in *Sugar Busters!*).

Lest your vigilance wane on serving your children some of the forbidden foods, bolster your resolve by referring to the list of the medical problems caused by childhood obesity on page 54 and remember that those same problems associated with obesity also apply to you and your spouse. If you help them remain slim and healthy, you will spare them the emotional trauma of being ostracized or treated cruelly, as are so many children who become obese.

We all want our children to live long and healthy lives. Analysis of 3,457 participants in the Framingham study reported in *Annals of Internal Medicine* indicate that overweight forty-year-old males and females lost seven years off their life expectancy, and obese females lost 5.8 years.[3] And remember, nearly 80 percent of fat children become fat adults!

# 7 | Digestion and Metabolism

The digestion and metabolism of the foods we eat are the keys to success in maintaining good nutrition and normal body weight. Because "we are what we eat," this is an important chapter for the proper understanding of our diet concept. It will provide you with a basic understanding of these processes so that you can maximize your gains in achieving these goals. This book is being written for a broad (pun intended!) audience, including health care professionals, so we will use some technical terms from time to time. As mentioned, if you come to a term you do not understand, please look it up in the Glossary.

## Digestion

Digestion encompasses the entire process from the time food is eaten until it is finally absorbed by the intestinal cells and sent on its way to the liver for metabolism. The most important aspect of digestion is the breakdown of proteins, fats, and carbohydrates into successively smaller units that can then be absorbed into the bloodstream and lymphatics to be used by the body in different ways.

Before any of this can happen, an integral part of the digestive process is the mixing and the churning (much like a concrete mixer) that occurs in the stomach. This process allows foods to be softened and mixed with fluid and be subjected to the initial phases of digestion. This mixing finally culminates in the gradual emptying of material from the stomach into the small intestine. Liquids empty from the stomach fairly quickly, within minutes, but solids empty much more slowly. The time that it takes for half of the stomach's solid contents to empty is somewhere between thirty and sixty minutes.

Smaller solid particles empty before larger ones in a very orderly, sequential fashion. The last solids to empty are fiber or indigestible solids, such as those found in leafy vegetables. When your mother advised, "Chew your food well," she was instinctively telling you the right thing to do because the smaller the particles, the more quickly the food would clear your stomach and, perhaps, avoid that uncomfortable feeling of fullness or the onset of indigestion. On the other hand, the more slowly the stomach empties, and food is absorbed in the small intestine, the more slowly the blood sugar rises and the insulin peaks.

Stomach emptying can be delayed by many external factors, including the types of foods eaten. A meal containing a large amount of fat can significantly delay stomach emptying, as can the drinking of large amounts of alcohol prior to, or with, the meal. While this may lower somewhat the glycemic result, slow or delayed stomach emptying can lead to the reflux of stomach contents—by this time usually very acidic—into the lower esophagus, causing heartburn, chest discomfort, fullness, and even nausea and vomiting. Many of us can recall these problems after a late evening of dining and drinking and going to bed with a full stomach! The moral is not to overconsume the fats, alcohols, or fruits in the first place.

As this stomach mix is gradually emptied into the small intestine, the breakdown of foods for absorption by our bodies begins in earnest. In the first part of the small intestine, called the duodenum, bile from the gallbladder and enzymes from the pancreas mix with the stomach contents and speed the breakdown of the different foods into smaller and smaller units. This mix moves farther down the small intestine where absorption takes place by the cells lining the intestine.

It is important to point out that the mixing of certain foods can have tremendous implications later on as these smaller units become absorbed. For instance, eating foods containing a modest amount of insoluble fiber can affect the rate of digestion and absorption of carbohydrates, thus causing these carbohydrates to have a much lower insulin-stimulating effect than if eaten by themselves. This would obviously be a good thing for the body.

Fruits eaten by themselves also are digested and absorbed at better rates than if eaten together with other carbohydrates and fats. The negative effect that eating fruits at the wrong time can have on the other foods in the digestive process is covered in Chapter 10.

## *Metabolism*

To *metabolize* essentially means "to change" and it entails the many processes that transform the nutrients in food to chemical substances that can be used by our bodies. The entire process is obviously quite complex. Metabolic rates often vary from person to person. This means that weight gain or loss for two people on the identical diet can vary considerably.

Although the process is complex, you should know that the liver plays the central role in the metabolism of foods, including alcohol, and in the metabolism of the majority of medications. So it is easy to see the importance of the liver in our nutritional well-being, and it behooves us all to take very good care of it because medical science cannot yet duplicate its functions. When the liver goes, it is "Adios, amigo!"

Now let's talk about what types of food get metabolized for use by our bodies. Everything we eat is either carbohydrates, which are broken down to simple sugar, 80 percent glucose and the rest fructose or galactose depending on whether we have had fruit or dairy products; proteins, which are broken down to amino acids; fats, which are broken down to triglycerides; and fiber, which is cellulose and cannot be broken down further. Of these four substances, only three are absorbed from our digestive tracts: sugars, amino acids, and triglycerides.

## Carbohydrates

Carbohydrates can be found in both plant and animal food sources. The overwhelming majority of the carbohydrates we eat are in the form of sugars and starches. Carbohydrates can be classified as simple sugars or more complex sugars, such as starch.

All carbohydrates absorbed by the body are eventually converted to glucose. Glucose is the body's main fuel, much like the gasoline that is put in a car. Glucose is either used immediately to provide energy or stored in the form of glycogen in the liver and in muscle to be utilized later. Any remaining glucose then is stored as fat.

In understanding the metabolism of carbohydrates and how this relates to our recommendations for good nutrition and weight loss, it is very important to think of carbohydrates in terms of how much of a peak or rise of glucose they can cause within the body when eaten. This can be more simply called the glycemic potential, which varies for different types of carbohydrates and in more scientific terms can be defined as the glycemic index. The glycemic index graph in Figure 7 (page 64) simply reflects the area under the curve representing the rise in blood sugar over a given time. Glucose has been assigned a relative value of 100 as its glycemic index, and the values of other carbohydrates are simply related to this level. Some substances actually have a higher glycemic potential than glucose! You will see more on the importance of a carbohydrate's glycemic potential later.

When the blood glucose level drops lower than it should be, glycogen, which is glucose in its stored form in the body, is broken down into glucose to raise the level of glucose and maintain a normal blood sugar level.

Carbohydrates, such as starches, which have a more complex structure, can, contrary to some commonly held beliefs, be digested and absorbed nearly as fast as the more simple carbohydrates, such as table sugar. When a carbohydrate is eaten, there is a rise in the level of blood glucose commensurate with the type and amount of carbohydrate ingested (i.e., higher for sugar, lower for fresh fruit). This rise in blood sugar (glucose) is then followed by the release of insulin, which causes a fall in the level of glucose primarily as it is driven into the cells of the body where it can be utilized as instant fuel or stored mainly as fat. Following this, the glucose level returns to its normal baseline.

### Figure 7.
# Glycemic index graph.

X=High-glycemic carbohydrate; O=Low-glycemic
carbohydrate.

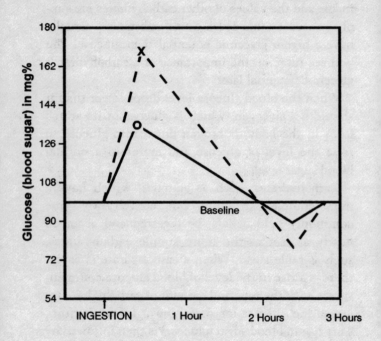

## *Proteins*

Proteins, the sources of which are meats, nuts, dairy products, and some vegetables, are made of subunits called amino acids. These amino acids are released from the protein by the action of enzymes secreted by the pancreas. Without these enzymes, protein molecules would not be absorbed because they are too large and complex to enter the bloodstream. Fortunately, in cases where pancreatic enzymes are missing, they can be provided in capsule form that can be taken with meals to aid the digestive process.

An average adult should consume per day *at least* one gram of protein for each kilogram (2.2 pounds) of weight, or somewhere between 55 and 70 grams (2 to 2.5 ounces) for the average man or woman.

Because there are both animal and vegetable sources of proteins and neither of these sources provides all of the amino acids that the body needs, a diet should be well balanced to provide both sources of protein.

Once proteins have been broken down into amino acids, they can be absorbed from the intestine and metabolized by the liver. Then, in general, amino acids can either be used by the body as the basic building blocks of all proteins, which make up all cells, hormones, and neurotransmitters (substances that relay signals in the nervous system), or amino acids can be converted into glucose, or sugar, by the liver through a process called *gluconeogenesis*, which is the manufacture of glucose from noncarbohydrate food sources, such as protein. The body's ability to manufacture its own glucose is important for maintaining normal energy requirements during periods of low-carbohydrate consumption, as glucose is the main fuel the body uses to meet its energy requirements.

## Fats

Fats, or lipids, are complex molecules composed of fatty acids and are derived from both animal and vegetable origins. Fats must be digested through the actions of pancreatic enzymes called lipases; otherwise, they cannot enter the body to any great extent and are passed in the stool. Even after fats are broken down into subunits, most of these remain insoluble in water and require a special type of absorption. Bile from the liver, which is stored in the gallbladder, plays a very important role in this absorption of fats by emulsifying or dissolving them. This is akin to using soap or any detergent to help in dissolving an oily substance. Without this process, fat subunits would be too large to enter the bloodstream from the intestine.

Some individuals who lack pancreatic enzymes must take enzymes with their food. Fats are absorbed through the intestinal tract as glycerols and are reconstituted while still in the intestinal wall as triglycerides that then enter the lymphatic system where these fats can be used by all the body's cells.

Cells use fat as fuel for energy production, as an important component of cell structures, and as a source of many essential substances manufactured by cells. An important function of fat that no one likes to think of is to provide insulation in the form of a layer of fat immediately underneath the skin. This should be only a thin layer, however, and it is almost always a source of constant restructuring in modern man and woman's attempts to control weight and body shape.

Cholesterol is not what most people think. Contrary to common belief, cholesterol is not a fat and has nothing to do with saturated fats. It is a compound belonging to a family of substances called *sterols*. Cholesterol can combine with fat as it circulates in the bloodstream to be distributed to all cells. Cholesterol is a vital substance in the formation of steroids, bile acids, hormones, and other substances.

Because cholesterol is so important, the body must provide a constant supply of cholesterol to the cells. Therefore, the body not only takes in cholesterol from food but also manufactures it, primarily in the liver. The liver can provide enough cholesterol to meet the body's needs even if a person were to take in no cholesterol in food!

Cholesterol manufactured in the liver circulates as lipoproteins for delivery to the cells. It is during this circulation in the bloodstream that cholesterol can be deposited on major arterial walls, especially at points of irritation, roughness, or small breaks in the lining of these vessels. This is the process referred to as *arteriosclerosis*, and it is the underlying process leading to coronary heart disease and in some cases hypertension (high blood pressure).

Now you know how your digestive system works and some of the things that help or hinder its efficiency. We keep mentioning and hinting at the importance of insulin. The next chapter is dedicated to helping you better understand the insulin connection.

# 8 | Insulin

You may ask, "Why do I want to know more about insulin?" It is just another seven-letter hormone. Insulin is the maestro, the conductor, the chief. It is the mission control system for metabolism. We must understand the actions of insulin to understand why the diet works.

Ready for some additional technical, but hopefully interesting, information? Banting and Best discovered insulin in 1921. This hormone is manufactured and secreted by the beta cells of the pancreas. The human pancreas stores about two hundred units of insulin. Normal people secrete about twenty-five to thirty units of insulin daily. Insulin is like a broom. It sweeps glucose, amino acids, and free fatty acids into cells where potential energy is stored as fat and glycogen to be used later.

In normal individuals, blood sugar levels do not vary much because of the harmonious and compensating hormonal actions of insulin and glucagon. Insulin is the only hormone that can prevent sugar (glucose) from rising to dangerously high levels.

Glucagon, also secreted by the pancreas, prevents the blood sugar from falling too low (to hypoglycemic levels).

Whereas insulin has been referred to as the hormone of feasting, glucagon is the hormone of fasting (or starvation). The main role of glucagon in humans appears to be the prevention of hypoglycemia (low blood glucose or blood sugar) by causing the normal breakdown of glycogen in the liver to form glucose. It also causes gluconeogenesis, which is the conversion of muscle protein to blood sugar.

Gluconeogenesis can occur during periods of starvation or excessive exercise. During the first twenty-four hours of fasting, glycogen in the liver is utilized, and then the body will begin using up muscle proteins. Glucagon secretion is stimulated by hypoglycemia, fasting, and also by the ingestion of a protein-rich meal.

Individuals can survive without glucagon, as in cases where the pancreas, which is the only known source of glucagon and insulin, is removed. A person must have insulin to survive, and this can be accomplished through insulin injections. Of course, removing the pancreas causes diabetes, often with wide swings in the blood sugar levels. Insulin given by injections is not as efficient in providing a continuous supply in exactly the right amount as is the pancreas.

After a person eats carbohydrates, the digestive enzymes break down the food. The blood in the intestines, having absorbed these simplified food substances, now has an elevated glucose level. This stimulates the release of insulin. As we have previously learned, insulin causes the storage of fat. When the blood sugar level falls too low, glucagon is secreted, which mobilizes stored fat into glucose, which raises blood sugar back to its normal level.

Glucose is the major stimulus for insulin secretion. Fructose, a sugar from fruits, and amino acids (proteins) from meats, cause a significant release of insulin only in the presence of previously elevated blood sugar. The overweight person probably has increased insulin production because of excessive stimulation of the pancreas through overeating and the development of, or genetic tendency toward, insulin resistance.

The increased insulin level then promotes the storage of sugar as glycogen in both the liver and muscle. After proteins and fats are ingested, insulin promotes the storage of protein in muscle and fat in fat cells as triglycerides. Insulin also prevents the breakdown of glycogen and triglycerides (fat). No wonder it is difficult to lose weight in the presence of elevated insulin levels.

Scientific literature documents that even low levels of circulating insulin inhibit fat breakdown.[1] The metabolic pathways involving insulin are exquisitely sensitive in causing the storage of fat and inhibiting its breakdown for use by the body.

Insulin further activates an enzyme, lipoprotein

lipase (enzymes are proteins that speed up metabolic actions), which promotes the removal of triglycerides from the bloodstream and their deposition in fat cells. Insulin also inhibits hormone-sensitive lipase (another enzyme) that breaks down stored fats. The net result of these two activities is an increase in stored fat that results in weight gain and an increase of abdominal girth.

Also adding to fat storage is the conversion of some of the sugar present in the blood. A percentage of the blood sugar is taken up by fat cells and, under the influence of our old friend insulin, is converted to still more fat. For our scientific readers, this involves glycerol 3-phosphate and free fatty acids. Insulin is a major deterrent to fat breakdown and a major facilitator of fat storage.

Insulin resistance is a condition of decreased responsiveness to insulin wherein the fat cells, liver cells, and muscle cells have become insensitive to normal levels of circulating insulin. Usually a small burst of insulin will lower blood sugar. However, in an insulin-resistant individual, this does not occur, and more insulin is required to do the job.

Obesity is the most common result of insulin resistance. Another frequently seen result of insulin resistance is Type 2 diabetes (non-insulin-dependent diabetes). In most Type 2 diabetics the circulating insulin levels and blood sugars are elevated, as are the blood cholesterol levels.

Obese individuals without diabetes usually have

elevated insulin levels with normal blood sugar levels. Unfortunately, the obese person with an elevated insulin level is probably on his way to developing diabetes. The pancreas may simply become exhausted from constant stimulation by glucose (sugar) and finally fail, resulting in diabetes. Diabetes is discussed specifically in Chapter 13.

Insulin promotes the storage of all food groups: glucose (carbohydrates), amino acids (proteins), and triglycerides (fats). These stored foods are available for use as an energy source later in a fasting state or simply between meals. The fall in insulin levels during fasting allows the breakdown of stored fat and stored sugar (glycogen). Fats and glycogen are then used as energy sources between meals.

As mentioned, obese people have elevated insulin levels in both the fasting and fed states. Lipoprotein lipase levels also are elevated in the obese. The enzyme, lipoprotein lipase, is important in the storage of fat. You now can see that obese individuals are metabolically ready at all times to store whatever they eat.

Again, it is no wonder that the obese person with an elevated insulin level has a hard time losing weight. But think of the benefits of a diet for this very same person that requires the presence of very little insulin in the system. We are now gaining on the answer to how to lose weight and improve our blood chemistry at the same time.

Syndrome X, described by Dr. G. M. Reaven, is a

combination of two or more of the following conditions: insulin resistance with resulting elevated insulin levels, elevated lipids (especially triglycerides), obesity, coronary artery disease, and hypertension. Insulin resistance probably is the most important part of this syndrome because in fact it often causes the other problems to occur. A significant number of patients with Syndrome X develop coronary artery disease and experience an increased number of fatal heart attacks.[2]

How about some good news? Fifty percent or more of insulin resistance can be reduced or even reversed as insulin resistance does not totally depend on our inherited genes. How can we decrease insulin levels or reduce insulin resistance? You are right! It is the SUGAR BUSTERS! way of eating. First, we must eat less of the particularly insulin-stimulating carbohydrates (high-glycemic carbohydrates). This helps with weight loss and, combined with exercise and smoking cessation, provides major nonmedical ways to accomplish this reduction of circulating insulin. Therefore, by lowering the insulin levels and decreasing insulin resistance, the incidence of obesity and probably the progression of heart disease will decrease.

Many people with coronary artery disease have similar body shapes. They are fatter in the abdomen, have beer bellies, and are thinner in the hips and buttocks. This is called central obesity (apple shape). Individuals with diabetes and insulin resistance have similar apple shapes, as opposed to pear shapes, where the fat is distributed in the hips and buttocks.

Dr. Wolever and coworkers in 1992 studied the benefits of a low-glycemic index diet in overweight non-insulin-dependent diabetics. They found a 7 percent drop in cholesterol after only six weeks.[3] Dr. Jenkins studied a low-glycemic (low-sugar) diet fed to normal males. After two weeks the men's cholesterol dropped an average of 15 percent, and insulin secretion dropped an amazing 32 percent![4]

After ingestion of 50 to 100 grams of glucose during a high-sugar meal, insulin levels usually become very elevated and can remain elevated for several hours. Eating high-carbohydrate (high-glycemic) meals three times a day and at bedtime can cause insulin to be elevated for eighteen out of twenty-four hours. The pancreas needs a rest, and so do fat cells. Imagine insulin pushing fat into cells eighteen hours a day. Only a few hours a day would be left for fat breakdown and fat loss. Fat would tend to accumulate at essentially all other times, resulting in you know what going you know where!

Understanding insulin and metabolism will now enable us to follow a healthier diet. As mentioned, not all carbohydrates are equal in their ability to stimulate insulin release. Carbohydrates that stimulate the most insulin secretion are called high-glycemic carbohydrates. Conversely, low-glycemic carbohydrates do not stimulate as much insulin secretion.

In 1981 Dr. David Jenkins published an article on the glycemic indexes of foods in the American Journal of Clinical Nutrition. He and others have since provided many additional measurements on the glycemic indexes of many common carbohydrates. Because you have learned the need to dodge the carbohydrates with the high-glycemic indexes, you can see why we provided you with some additional glycemic index formation. Figure 3 (pages 25–30) lists the glycemic indexes for many of our most commonly consumed carbohydrates.

## 9 | The Sugar Busters! Concept

*Sugar Busters!* is a nutritional lifestyle, not just another fad diet. It is about how, what, and when to eat and, yes, it does involve exercise. You will find *Sugar Busters!* logical, practical, and reasonable and you will not be burdened by having to weigh, count, and measure. Because we encourage you to avoid refined sugar and processed grain products, *Sugar Busters!* will be a "less" sugar diet but definitely not a "no" sugar diet. In fact we strongly encourage you to make a commitment to choosing correct carbohydrates, those low-insulin-producing carbohydrates. Insulin causes you to convert and store excess sugar as fat and also store excess fat as fat. You cannot live without insulin, but you can live much better without too much insulin. Remember, most of the fat on your body comes from sugar, not fat.

Modulating insulin secretion is the key to our *Sugar Busters!* diet. Successfully controlling insulin through nutrition will allow you to improve your performance and health through nutrition. To control insulin you must control the intake of sugar, both the refined variety and the kind so abundant and stimulative in many carbohydrates.

We recommend selecting foods in forms that stimulate insulin secretion in a more deliberate, controlled manner rather than those that cause the immediate outpouring of this hormone. Eating in this way will result in lower average insulin levels in our blood throughout any given period. This in turn has a markedly beneficial effect on reducing fat synthesis and storage, as well as curbing the harmful effects that too much insulin has on the cardiovascular system.

Because insulin is the key to our concept, carbohydrates become the cornerstone. The basic building block of all carbohydrates is sugar. Sugar absorbed from our digestive tract into our blood then stimulates insulin secretion to assist in the transport of sugar into cells as an energy source. The type of the ingested carbohydrate ultimately affects the rate of sugar absorption and, therefore, insulin secretion.

Refined sugar and processed grain products, stripped of their coatings or husks, are almost immediately absorbed in a very concentrated fashion, resulting in rapid rise in blood sugar followed by secretion of large quantities of insulin. This is the case with most candies, cookies, cakes, pies, and pastries. A diet of refined sugar and processed grain products, therefore, produces a rather marked elevation in average insulin levels throughout a twenty-four-hour period. The additional insulin is then available to promote fat deposition as well as many other previously discussed undesirable effects

However, carbohydrates in an unrefined form, such as fruits, green vegetables, dried beans, and whole grains, require further digestion alteration before absorption. This in turn causes a proportionate reduction in the rate and quantity of insulin secretion—a modulation of insulin secretion. The end result is lower average insulin levels and less fat synthesis, storage, and weight gain as well as fat breakdown. The positive effects on our appearance and cardiovascular system become apparent.

The *Sugar Busters!* lifestyle involves eating high fiber vegetables and whole grains. The fiber in both of these food products has a beneficial effect on your digestive process and overall health. Fruits are encouraged on *Sugar Busters!* and are excellent as snacks. Meats are an important source of protein but should be lean and trimmed. *Sugar Busters!* is cautious about fat. We encourage reduced fat products when choosing milk and cheese and strongly advocate careful attention to saturated fats. Too much saturated fat and trans fats, those oils used in fast food establishments, are very harmful not only to your waistline but also to your heart and blood vessels.

Hydration is important and everyone is encouraged to drink six to eight glasses of water daily.

Missing meals is not healthy. It is important to eat three regular meals daily, and appropriate snacks are allowed. But moderation in portion size is also important. If you are not careful you easily can eat too much of even a correct food choice. Late night snacking is not allowed. Eating at night before going to bed only raises your insulin level and encourages cholesterol production since most cholesterol is manufactured while you are sleeping.

Exercise is an important part of any successful nutritional lifestyle. You should strive to exercise at least twenty minutes four days per week so that you will raise your resting heart rate. However, most people are over-ambitious about exercise, and when they do not meet their expectations they just don't do it at all. They literally bite off more (exercise) than they can chew (perform). A little exercise will go a long way and a little certainly is better than none at all (see Chapter 17).

*Sugar Busters!* is not restrictive. You can eat from all food groups, but we encourage you to make the best selections within each food group. *Sugar Busters!* is not an extreme or radical approach to nutrition but rather the voice of moderation. A great plan not followed yields poor results. *Sugar Busters!* has been developed to encourage compliance rather than cheating. The closer you follow *Sugar Busters!* the better your results.

Likewise, lean meats are important to our nutritional well-being. Not only do they supply much-

**Figure 8.**
**Deaths from cancer, heart disease, strokes, and accidents.**

Source: Modified from Marmot and Brunner (1991).

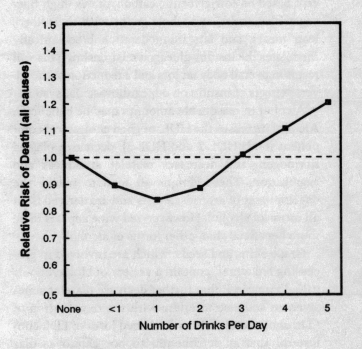

needed protein, the building blocks of our bodies, but also ingested protein stimulates glucagon secretion. Glucagon, also from the pancreas, promotes the breakdown of stored fat, creating a "fat loss" for our bodies.

The picture should now become clear. A diet concept based on low-glycemic carbohydrates (high-fiber vegetables, fruits, and whole grains with their fiber), lean meats, and fats in moderation biochemically modulates the insulin–glucagon relationship. This will result in overall body fat loss and a reduction of the adverse effects of insulin on our cardiovascular system.

Alcohol in reasonable amounts may be beneficial. Alcohol increases the HDL, or good cholesterol component (both HDL-2 and HDL-3), decreases plasma fibrinogen, and decreases platelet stickiness and aggregation. These actions all tend to reduce the development of arteriosclerosis and are derived from all forms of alcohol. However, red wine appears to be more beneficial than other forms of alcohol.

Grape skins and seeds, which are involved in processing red wines, contain a variety of bioflavonoids called vitamin P that further decrease platelet adhesiveness and also interfere with the oxygenation of LDL cholesterol. It is the oxidized form of LDL cholesterol that is detrimental to our cardiovascular systems.

The curve for the relationship between alcohol consumption and mortality is U-shaped and is shown in Figure 8, page 81. In moderation there is a potential benefit to our cardiovascular system, but in excess the curve changes quickly to the detriment of the consumer. Therefore, responsible use of alcohol is a must.

But, contrary to conventional wisdom, alcohol is responsible for considerably more health-related problems than even tobacco. An aspirin a day, coupled with eating red or green grapes, can more safely impart to our bodies all the beneficial effects ascribed to alcohol consumption.

We believe the problem of obesity in the United States has been caused by the population adhering to the government's recommended food pyramid. We propose the pyramid in Appendix A.

You have now completed the more technical portion of our book, and although we cannot award you with an M.D. in digestion, metabolism, or cardiology, you should be much better equipped to understand the more practical suggestions on eating for good health and weight loss that follow. The conversations with your own doctors and nutritionists or dietitians also should become more interesting!

In summary, the basis of our concept is to have a positive influence on insulin and glucagon secretion through nutrition. This is achieved by eating a diet composed of natural unrefined sugars, whole unprocessed grains, vegetables, fruits, lean meats, fiber, and alcohol (if any) in moderation. You and your family deserve the best. Make the correct nutritional choice and join the *Sugar Busters!* lifestyle.

# 10 | Eating Patterns

All successful nutritional concepts involve the "what," "why," "when," and "how." In the preceding chapters we have discussed the "what" (low sugar) and "why" (regulate insulin secretion), but now we need to address the "when" and "how" that will bring everything together into three full meals and an occasional snack. For many of you, success on the *Sugar Busters!* lifestyle will require changing your current eating habits.

More frequent smaller meals stimulate less overall insulin secretion than one or two large meals, because long intervals between meals will alter the body's response to insulin secretion and increase fat storage. Therefore, we should strive to consume at least three balanced meals every day.

Some studies indicate that eating as many as six small meals a day may provide even better control of the insulin response and even help in lowering cholesterol. While we have no problem with this eating pattern, we believe many people will find it impractical to fit this into their daily schedules.

As discussed in Chapter 29 ("Myths") it is not necessary to count calories. In addition, it is not necessary to count sugar grams, fat grams, or protein grams. Not only is trying to do this frustrating, but the results are almost always unreliable. Your daily dietary intake should consist of high-fiber carbohydrates, lean meats as sources of protein, and primarily unsaturated fats. The *Sugar Busters!* plan makes a point of limiting saturated fat.

Portion size is very important. Don't overfill your plate—your meat and vegetables should fit nicely in the center of the plate and not extend onto or over the rim. If you place proper servings on the plate, then the need to count grams is not necessary. Remember, once you have filled your plate appropriately, do not go back for seconds or thirds—this will prevent you from eating too much of an otherwise glycemically acceptable carbohydrate.

In addition, because most cholesterol is manufactured at night, when we are sleeping, a large meal of any type should not be eaten just before going to bed. You should try to finish your evening meal by approximately 8:00 P.M. Once dinner is over, the kitchen is closed—no midnight snacks! Following this advice also should reduce or even eliminate most of the indigestion or heartburn that can awaken us in the middle of the night.

Appropriate snacks are encouraged, and most fruits (except watermelons, pineapple, raisins, and ripe bananas, which have a high glycemic index) are ideal for this occasion. Some individuals who experience frequent indigestion may benefit from eating fruit thirty minutes before or two hours after a meal. Fruit is digested primarily in the small intestine, and when eaten with other solids, its emptying from the stomach is delayed. This permits fermentation that produces indigestion (heartburn) and often gas (bloating).

Most fruits contain the basic sugar fructose which stimulates approximately one-third of the insulin secretion as an equal amount of sucrose (table sugar). Consequently, fruit alone as a snack is very beneficial, but in combination with other carbohydrates loses the advantage of lower insulin secretion that is achieved when eaten by itself. However, fruit juice may be consumed prior to a meal, such as breakfast, because fluid empties more quickly from the stomach than solids, especially if the juice is drunk first.

In general, fluids should be drunk in small quantities during meals. Washing food down with lots of fluids can cause us to skip over the step of proper chewing, necessary to break food into smaller, more appropriate particles for better digestion. Excess fluid with meals also dilutes the digestive juices, which reduces their ability to thoroughly interact with food not only in the mouth but also in the stomach. This may result in partially digested food entering the small intestine, which can cause cramping.

Fluids may be consumed between meals. But be careful because most sodas and even popular sports drinks are loaded with sugar, and some also contain large quantities of caffeine. Overconsumption of regular coffee and tea also can present the problem of too much caffeine. Caffeine makes the stomach produce gastric acid, which stimulates, not suppresses, appetite. Water and decaffeinated drinks, without added sugar, are preferable. You should make a conscientious effort to drink six to eight glasses of water a day. This is beneficial to the proper function of many of your organs, especially the kidneys. Water consumed throughout the day will lessen your desire for food, thereby helping in weight control.

Alcoholic beverages present a slightly different problem. Alcohol consumed with food (on a full stomach) is absorbed more slowly, which causes less insulin secretion and potentially less intoxicating effects. Therefore, if you choose to consume alcohol, do so on a full stomach and only in reasonable quantities. As a word of caution, mixers for drinks usually contain a lot of sugar, as does beer (which contains maltose), so neither is considered appropriate for a healthy diet. A dry (low-sugar) red wine is the preferred alcoholic beverage.

Some diets have recommended against mixing certain carbohydrates, such as pasta and rice, with protein. These combinations supposedly stimulate the secretion of competing digestive enzymes. We believe the problem is not so much the carbohydrate-protein combination as the type of carbohydrate that is consumed. For example, a meal of meatballs (without added sugar) and whole-grain spaghetti is allowed. As the list in Chapter 2 indicates, modest quantities of most unrefined or unprocessed carbohydrates are acceptable. Of course, starches in most forms (except sweet potatoes, which contain a considerable amount of fiber) are harmful and should not be eaten alone or in combination with other foods. Sorry, no potatoes with your meal, except for sweet potatoes!

Shoppers beware! Even the best intentions can go awry. Producers of foods have made it difficult for us to eat healthily. Most breakfast cereals, although advertised as being the best product for your health, are laced with either white sugar, brown sugar, molasses, corn syrup, or honey. In fact, it is difficult to purchase a pure natural-grain cereal. They do exist, but to find them you must closely read the fine print on the side of the box. The same problem applies to bottled, canned, or other packaged foods, sauces, and dressings. Almost all of them have significant amounts of added sugar. Of course, fresh vegetables are your healthiest choice, followed by those that are quick-frozen and those canned without added sugars.

Whole-grain breads, rolls, muffins, and other products are available in most large or specialty grocery stores. But you must be careful that our old nemesis, sugar, has not been added in one form or another. When we really begin to look at what we are eating, we quickly realize just how much sugar is present in almost everything we have been eating. To remind you where this has gotten us, refer to Figure 4 (page 33).

As you now begin to select foods and plan your meals and snacks, remember that sugar and high-glycemic-index carbohydrates are what you need to avoid. While sugar stimulates insulin secretion, which instructs our body to create and hold fat, protein stimulates glucagon secretion, which does just the opposite. Glucagon helps instruct our body to mobilize fat and convert it back to glucose, which reduces our fat stores and waistlines.

A diet that reduces insulin secretion while enhancing glucagon secretion is the most beneficial. This method of eating reduces body fat and cholesterol as well as the many health problems caused by both of them. Therefore, good dietary sources of protein are a must. All lean, trimmed meats, such as beef, fish, and fowl, are recommended. These should be grilled, baked, or broiled, since frying often involves saturated fats, trans fats, and/or a batter made with refined flour. Other excellent and healthy protein sources are eggs, cheese, and nuts. Remember, it is not necessarily the fat you eat but the fat you create from sugar that is ruining your appearance and health.

You should now be getting hungry for what you really like but previously thought you should not eat. Light the grill, and let's see what's for dinner. Chapter 11 lists a huge variety of acceptable foods and Chapter 21 outlines a lifetime meal plan to help you on your way to a successful *Sugar Busters!* lifestyle.

# 11 | Acceptable Foods and Substitutes

The bottom line of any diet is to choose the proper things to eat. In this chapter we hope to give you advice and examples to make these choices easy. In addition, we will briefly comment on caffeine, artificial sweeteners, and the spices that are part of our everyday diet.

But first, let's look at some notable exceptions that probably will surprise you. "Potatoes are for pigs and corn is for cattle"—so say the French, and with good reason. These foods fatten these animals just as they fatten us. Potatoes, beets, and many other root vegetables are simply starch, a storage form of glucose. Once inside our digestive tracts, they are quickly converted to pure sugar. Their absorption is rapid, and the resulting insulin response is very significant.

How many of us, for the sake of dieting, have not eaten a tender, juicy steak but instead have opted for a baked potato? If we scooped out a baked potato and filled most of the skin with sugar, would you eat it? Certainly not! However, that is essentially what you are doing when you eat a baked potato, because it is quickly converted to sugar in your stomach.

Hybrid corn that has large, fleshy kernels also causes a rapid insulin response. Maize, the original Indian corn, has smaller kernels and more fiber, and therefore has a much more moderate absorption and insulin release. Many Native Americans became overtly diabetic when they altered their diets and started eating the modern hybrid variety of corn,[1] which has a greater sugar load.

So to the list of foods to avoid, which already includes refined sugar and processed grain products, especially white bread and white rice, now add potatoes, beets, corn, and too many carrots. This may seem a little discouraging, but in fact the list of *recommended* foods is quite extensive. Let's see what we can eat and enjoy (Figure 9, pages 93–95), as well as what we should avoid (Figure 10, pages 95–96).

In stores in America it is extremely difficult to find many packaged or canned foods without one or more added sugars. Also, beware of sauces, such as catsups and most barbecue sauces, that are laced with added sugars. Most commercial salad dressings contain one or more forms of sugar as well.

Last, remember that even with moderate- and low-glycemic-index foods such as beans and sweet potatoes, you cannot expect to eat three or four portions of these foods at a meal and not gain or retain weight! It all adds up, so keep an eye on your total consumption.

**Figure 9.**
# Acceptable Foods

## Meats

| | | |
|---|---|---|
| Lean beef* | Chicken* | Pheasant |
| Lamb* | Turkey* | Partridge |
| Pork* | Quail | Elk |
| Veal* | Venison | Dove |
| Antelope | Fish | Duck* |
| Rabbit | Shellfish | |
| Goose* | | |
| Alligator | | |

## Vegetables

| | |
|---|---|
| Beans | Squash |
| Lentils | Zucchini |
| Peas | Mushrooms |
| Spinach | Asparagus |
| Turnip greens | Artichokes |
| Collard greens | Lettuce |
| Hearts of palm | Okra |
| Watercress | Carrots, in moderation |
| Cabbage | Celery |
| Cauliflower | Brussels sprouts |
| Broccoli | Dill pickles |
| Cucumbers | Radishes |
| Eggplant | Sweet potatoes |
| Mirliton (chayote) | Onions |
| Bell peppers | |

## Fruit

| | |
|---|---|
| Apples | Tangerines |
| Lemons | Oranges |
| Satsumas | Limes |
| Pears | Mangos |
| Cherries | Peaches |
| Berries | Dates |
| Kiwis | Honeydews |
| Apricots | Grapes |
| Grapefruits | Plums |
| Cantaloupes | Avocados |
| Tomatoes | Pumpkin |

## Dairy Products

| | |
|---|---|
| Milk | Yogurt |
| Cheese | Cream |
| Eggs | Butter |

## Grains and Cereals

Whole-grain products, including breads and
   pastas (without sucrose, dextrose, maltose,
   honey, molasses, brown sugar, or corn syrup)
Brown rice
Wheat bran
Oat bran
Other unrefined grains
Oatmeal

Miscellaneous
Nuts
Spices†
Garlic
Chocolate (60 percent or greater cocoa)
Tabasco sauce
Coffee‡
Tea‡
Sodas and other soft drinks with artificial
    sweeteners§
Fruit juices without added sugar
Olive oil, canola oil
Peanut butter without added sugar
Pure fruit jelly without added sugar

Notes:
* Trimmed or skinned.
† Spices are generally allowable but have little, if any, nutritional value.
‡ Most individuals should consume no more than two or three caffeinated beverages daily. Caffeine can cause cardiac irregularity, high blood pressure, increased gastric acid secretion, and increased appetite. However, sudden cessation of caffeine may produce temporary withdrawal symptoms, such as headache and irritability.
§ Artificial sweeteners are not harmful to the vast majority of individuals. However, they have no nutritional value.

## Figure 10.
## Foods to Avoid and Acceptable Substitutes

| Foods to Avoid | Acceptable Substitutes |
|---|---|
| Potatoes (red or white) | Beans, lentils, sweet potatoes, broiled tomatoes with cheese, mushrooms |

| Foods to Avoid | Acceptable Substitutes |
| --- | --- |
| White rice | Brown rice |
| Corn (including cornbread or corn meal products) | Okra, peas, asparagus, squash |
| Carrots (too many) | Spinach, kale, collard greens, broccoli |
| Beets | Hearts of palm, artichokes |
| White bread | Whole-grain breads without added sugars, whole-grain pasta |
| All refined sugar | Nutrasweet (aspartame) or other artificial sweeteners, stevia, Sweet Balance, fructose |
| Other refined products, such as cookies, cakes, and so on | Sugar-free ice cream, sugar-free yogurt, sugar-free vanilla ice cream, and diet root beer (occasionally) |

## 12 | Stocking and Unstocking the Pantry

Before you stock your pantry and refrigerator, you should first "unstock" the forbidden items. This is very important because it will eliminate the temptation near at hand, prevent your children or grandchildren from taking samples of fat-building foods, and make room for more wholesome things.

How much inventory one keeps is a personal choice. Following are suggestions for those who have a little room in the pantry and cook at home from time to time.

### Unstocking the Pantry

Get rid of the following:

White potatoes
White bread
White rice
White flour
Non-whole-grain pastas
Sugar-laden salad dressings and sauces

Jellies and jams containing added sugars (all-fruit products are okay in moderation)

Sugar, syrup, candy bars

Corn chips, potato chips

Crackers or wafers containing enriched flours

Canned goods with added sugars

Fruit juices containing added sugars

Sugar-sweetened soft drinks

Teriyaki sauces

## Stocking the Pantry

### Dry Pantry

Stone-ground whole wheat flour

Stone-ground whole rye flour

Whole oatmeal or steel-cut oats

Packets of Equal, Sweet 'N Low, fructose, or stevia

Whole-wheat pasta

No-sugar-added pasta sauce

Brown rice

Dry black, kidney, navy, or pinto beans

Dry lentils and peas

White, apple cider, and balsamic vinegar* (preferably only 1 or 2 percent sugar)

Sweet potatoes, yellow onions, garlic

---

* Vinegar lowers the GI of a meal

Assorted nuts, or bags of walnuts, almonds, pecans, or macadamia nuts

Olive oil and canola oil

Salad dressing with no sugar added

Natural peanut butter

Canned tuna, salmon, sardines

Canned mild green chilies

Salsa

Canned tomatoes

Tabasco sauce

Canned greens (spinach, mixed greens, kale, collards), beans (black, pinto, navy, kidney), other vegetables (green beans, peas, etc.)

Assorted spices of your choice plus Worcestershire, and soy sauces

Mustard

No-sugar-added mayonnaise

coffee, tea, green tea

## Refrigerator

Low-fat milk

Low-fat cream cheese

Cheese of your choice

Eggs

Low-fat sour cream

No-sugar-added yogurt

Butter

Romaine lettuce, fresh vegetables of your choice

## Freezer

Canadian bacon
Smoked ham hocks
Frozen greens (spinach, kale) and other vegetables (green beans, peas, broccoli, cauliflower)
No-sugar-added ice cream
Meat, poultry, or fish

## Fruits

Apples
Oranges
Peaches
Pears
Plums
Cantaloupe
Blueberries
Raspberries
Strawberries
Green bananas
Tomatoes
Blackberries

## 13 | Why <u>Sugar Busters!</u> Works for Diabetics

Everyone should read this chapter, not just those individuals with diabetes. We all have friends or relatives with diabetes. After you read this book, and particularly this chapter, you will be able to give those diabetics some intriguing advice that can help them eat in a way that will reduce their blood sugar levels and most likely their need for insulin or oral medication.

The American Diabetes Association and the U.S. Department of Health and Human Services has recognized that a large number of people in the United States have early symptoms of diabetes and that, left untreated, most of these people will go on to develop diabetes within ten years. These organizations are now using the term *pre-diabetes* to describe blood sugar levels that are higher than normal but not yet indicative of full-blown diabetes. They are also urging that people be screened for the presence of this condition.[1]

The two main categories of diabetes are *insulin-*

*dependent*, or *Type 1*, diabetes and *non-insulin-dependent*, or *Type 2*, diabetes (although many Type 2 diabetics ultimately become dependent on orally administered medication or injections of insulin to control their blood sugars). Another less common type of diabetes occurs during pregnancy. This is referred to as *gestational diabetes*, which we will discuss later in this chapter.

Over 90 percent of all patients with diabetes have Type 2 diabetes. Type 1 diabetics generally acquire the disease younger, are thinner, and require insulin injections. Type 2 diabetics have historically been older (over forty at the time of onset), obese, and initially could be treated with diet and exercise or diet and oral medications. However, the recent surge in Type 2 diabetes in children is changing the way we think about this form of the disease. Diet still is the most important treatment for all types of diabetes, and *Sugar Busters!* describes a way of eating that is particularly effective for all types of diabetes.

When we wrote this book we knew that the way of eating we described had to be helpful for diabetics. But the favorable responses from those diabetics who have followed the *Sugar Busters!* lifestyle exceeded our expectations. Many borderline Type 2 diabetics have seen their blood glucose drop back to within the normal range of 90 to 110 milligrams per deciliter (mg/dL). We have seen many Type 2 diabetics who require insulin improve to a point where injections are no longer needed.

The following is an example that typifies what this way of eating can do for a borderline diabetic. Joe Canizaro, an entrepreneur and prominent New Orleans developer, said, "In 1997 I had my annual physical, and upon completion of all the usual tests, my doctor said, 'Joe, what the heck have you been doing?' 'I don't know, Doc, what's wrong with me?' The doctor said, 'Nothing! I have been telling you for six years that you are a borderline diabetic, but this time your blood sugar is normal.' I said, 'Well, Doc, I've been trying a new way of eating I read about in a book called *Sugar Busters!*" We checked with Joe in late 2002 to see how he was doing. He said, "My blood sugar is still normal. I am not a borderline diabetic anymore."

A good example of success by a Type 2 diabetic who required oral medication for his diabetes is Dr. John Crisp, dean of the College of Engineering at the University of New Orleans. Dr. Crisp was given a copy of *Sugar Busters!* by the chancellor of the university, Dr. Gregory O'Brien, who was concerned about John's health. After following the way of eating recommended in *Sugar Busters!* Dr. Crisp found that he no longer needed any pills and that his quality of life had improved dramatically.

Let's now talk about the experience of Jerry Crowder, a retired executive from Houston, Texas. Jerry, seventy-two years old, was overweight and a full-fledged diabetic. Jerry was given a copy of our manuscript a month before the original *Sugar*

*Busters!* was published because we knew he was diabetic and believed that the *Sugar Busters!* lifestyle would be beneficial for him. Two months later, one of our authors saw Jerry and asked him, "How are you doing?" Jerry replied that he had lost thirty pounds, but what he really liked about our plan was that he was *off* insulin! He had started his injections with 28 units of Humulin N every morning for the past two and a half years, but his doctor said he no longer needed it. He said his doctor told him, "Jerry, your blood glucose was 240 when we started you on the insulin injections, but now it is only 128. You are only a borderline diabetic, and you no longer need these injections." Jerry told our author that he could even have a glass or two of wine in the evening without excessively elevating his blood sugar.

These are success stories! What does this mean for Jerry and all those like Joe and John and Jerry who are able to achieve similar results? If diabetics (most of whom, if not all, are insulin-resistant) can keep their blood sugar near normal by eating in a way that requires very little insulin secretion, they will dramatically reduce the process that causes deterioration of their vision, kidneys, nerves, and circulatory system.

Why is this diet so effective for diabetics? Either a diabetic's pancreas does not manufacture the correct amount of insulin or his or her body does not respond to the insulin in an efficient manner. Most often the culprit is insulin resistance. Insulin resistance means that one's body needs more insulin to maintain its blood sugar in a normal range than does the body of a non-diabetic person who has consumed exactly the same meal. Diabetics following the *Sugar Busters!* lifestyle will be less likely to be out of control than they would be on most other diabetic diets that do not differentiate, as we do, the good carbohydrates from the high-glycemic, insulin-demanding carbohydrates.

Diabetics frequently have damage to their kidneys, eyes, nerves, and cardiovascular system. Diminished circulation and nerve damage (neuropathy) may ultimately cause so much damage to the extremities that they have to be amputated. Injections of insulin, although designed to control elevated glucose in a Type 2 diabetic, often are inefficient. Injected insulin is delivered at predetermined rates that often do not exactly coincide with the requirement created by the consumption of differing amounts of various foods. A properly functioning pancreas in a body that utilizes insulin normally will secrete insulin into the bloodstream in precisely the required amounts at exactly the right time. This precision is not yet achievable with devices that mechanically deliver insulin. So a diabetic should not eat in a fashion that creates a big demand for insulin.

The most severe damage occurs most frequently in diabetics whose blood sugar levels remain the most out of balance. A diet low in refined sugar, white potatoes, and processed grain products does not cause gross elevation in blood sugars in the first place, so there is not as much exposure to organ damage.

We believe early intervention with a low-glycemic, high-fiber diet can prevent or significantly postpone the onset of this disease. If the diet is coupled with exercise, the chance of developing diabetes drops even more. (For additional information relative to the prevention of diabetes, see Chapter 5.)

Diabetes is a very common disease. Every year more and more cases of diabetes are diagnosed, and the percentage of the population having diabetes continues to increase. The highest rate of increase in the last decade has been in our *children*! (See Chapter 6.)

Diabetes has been found to be more prevalent in Afro-Americans, Native Americans, and Hispanics than in Caucasians. The rate of diagnosis for those who already have diabetes in these ethnic groups is also thought to lag behind the rest of the population. If you are in one of these groups, you should be very mindful of any risk factors for or early indicators of diabetes. These include being overweight or obese, having developed gestational diabetes during pregnancy (go back and ask your doctor), having a family history of diabetes, having elevated blood sugar, or having had an impaired glucose tolerance test.

The diabetes epidemic is a worldwide phenomenon. The common usage of refined sugars and now highly refined grain products and even French fries is a worldwide phenomenon. Over 100 million people in all countries have diabetes, and that number is estimated to grow to 250 million by 2015. The occurrence of diabetes increases with age and also with obesity for all groups (Figure 11, page 110).

The Pima Indians in the southwestern United States have the highest incidence of diabetes in the world.[2] When large-kernel hybridized corn was substituted for the traditional small-kernel, fibrous ears of corn, the rate of diabetes among the Pimas soared to 50 percent! The glycemic index of many of the Pima Indians' traditional foods was low compared to that of the hybridized corn and highly refined carbohydrates, and their bodies could not efficiently handle the increased sugar load.[3]

According to experts from at a recent meeting of the American Association of Clinical Endocrinologists as many as 50 percent of the people with undetected diabetes already have complications such as nerve damage, eye, kidney disease, or heart disease by the time the diabetes is detected.[4] Early screening is indeed wise.

We do not recommend that a diabetic eat any foods with a high glycemic load. While it is true that all carbohydrates are converted to glucose in our bodies, it just does not make sense for diabetics to put themselves at risk of unbalancing their blood sugar by consumption of foods that cause a rush of sugar into the bloodstream, such as candy and cake.

And we do not recommend these foods for nondiabetics, either, because they demand a large release of insulin from the pancreas and can result in weight gain. In some individuals, frequent consumption of such foods can eventually exhaust the pancreas, which will result in diabetes.

Relative to exercise, a ten-year Harvard University study of nearly 40,000 men found that those who watched the most TV, over 40 hours a week, had three times the risk of developing diabetes as the men who watched the least amount of TV.[5] The researchers reported that the avid TV watchers tended to exercise less and ate more red or processed meat, snacks, refined grains, and sweets; they also ate fewer fruits and vegetables and fewer whole grains. Again, the *Sugar Busters!* lifestyle can help move you out of harm's way.

**A strong word of caution:** If you are currently taking insulin or other diabetic medication and start the *Sugar Busters!* way of eating, consult your doctor because you will probably require less than your current dose of medication. It is very likely that you will not need as much insulin, and if you are a Type 2 diabetic who closely follows this diet, quite possibly none at all.

What about Type 1 diabetics, whose bodies do not manufacture much insulin? Does this diet work for them? Yes, it does help. By not eating meals rich in refined or processed carbohydrates (sugars), which create a large requirement for insulin,

Type 1 diabetics will not need as much insulin to keep their blood glucose in a normal range. A Type 1 diabetic will always require some amount of insulin; however, eating in this fashion promotes lower insulin requirements and is certainly healthier. Remember, our bodies did not evolve on diets that created a great need for high insulin levels, and the damage to our organs and circulatory system is most pronounced when our blood sugar is the most out of balance.

We previously mentioned gestational diabetes. Although gestational diabetes is temporary, it does indicate a strong tendency for the mother to be susceptible to Type 2 diabetes. Over time, 50 percent to 70 percent of gestational diabetics develop Type 2 diabetes. Those who are obese before or after pregnancy develop it at higher rates. Importantly, untreated gestational diabetes can have a major impact on the mother and, unfortunately, the unborn child, who will also stand a higher chance of becoming diabetic later in life. All pregnant women should be screened for gestational diabetes between the twenty-fourth and twenty-eighth weeks of pregnancy. A low-glycemic diet full of fruits and appropriate vegetables will help prevent pregnant women from gaining excess weight and developing gestational diabetes.

As illustrated in Figure 4, page 33, just fifteen hundred years ago refined sugar did not exist, and neither did the hybridized, plump, and juicy

Figure 11.

# Likelihood of developing diabetes within 10 years related to percent overweight at initial examination

Source: Reprinted with permission from Diabetes 1996: Vital Statistics, 1996, American Diabetes Association, Inc.

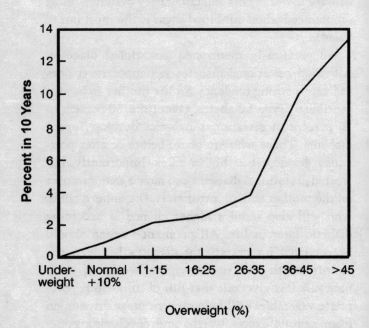

vegetables and grain products that have a much lower fiber content and a much higher glycemic index. Highly processed flours and grains, such as today's white rice, did not exist because the technology was not available to accomplish such complete refining and fiber removal. According to U.S. Department of Agriculture statistics (Figure 4, page 33), American food manufacturers are using an average of over 154 pounds of added refined sugar per person, per year (that is over one-third of a pound, or fifty-three teaspoons per day!) Add to that the consumption of large amounts of high-glycemic-index carbohydrates that we eat, and we have individuals with glucose overdose for their under-designed digestive systems.

Does consumption of refined sugar and highly refined carbohydrates cause or aggravate diabetes? It certainly does aggravate diabetes, and studies of large populations over many years strongly suggests that excess refined sugar and refined carbohydrate consumption is either directly or indirectly causing diabetes or at least speeding its onset by causing so many people to become obese and/or insulin-resistant.

Examination of data from the Harvard Nurses' Health Study by Dr. Jorge Salmerion et al. sounded a loud wake-up call about the risks associated with developing Type 2 diabetes.[6] That study of 65,173 previously healthy women, ages forty to sixty-five, found that the women who ate a high-glycemic and low-fiber diet had a 250 percent greater chance of developing diabetes than those who ate a low-glycemic, high-fiber diet. The study also recommended that diets should include minimally refined grains (as *Sugar Busters!* recommends). This type of diet is obviously a great way to help prevent diabetes. The conclusions from this world-renowned study have broken the backs of the critics who have said there was no value in using the glycemic index or glycemic load in helping to guide one's diet.

Let us examine other statistics. The rate of diabetes in the United States has more than tripled since 1958, which correlates closely with increased sugar consumption (Figure 4, page 33). What else are we consuming in amounts so different from what our recent forebears ate? Certainly not fat; the percentage of calories from fat in our diets has actually decreased since the late 1970s, from 40 percent to 34 percent; more important, the actual consumption per person per day is down from 85 grams to 73 grams (a 16 percent drop). Yet the incidence of obesity has doubled since the late 1970s, and on average people weigh eleven to twelve pounds more than when they were consuming larger quantities of fat!

What other products are we consuming at such an increasing rate than sugar? Sodas? Coffee? Well, sodas usually contain huge quantities of sugar (see

Chapter 19), so when you drink soda, you're just adding sugar to your diet. Does coffee cause diabetes or obesity? We don't think so. Coffee is not a problem unless you add large amounts of sugar or drink excessive amounts and get too much caffeine, which may cause other problems.

Because the rate of obesity in the United States for both children and adults has more than doubled since the 1960s (with most of the increase since 1980), and because sugar consumption has gone up another 20 percent just since 1980, what better correlation does anyone want between consumption of nutritionless refined sugar and what is causing us to get fat? Is not the answer to this dramatic increase in the rates of obesity and diabetes so blatantly obvious that it defies logic for everyone not to see it? How much more obvious can the connection between refined sugar consumption and obesity and diabetes get?

Add to this the fact that the correlation also makes physiological sense. Most people with diabetes were fat before they became diabetic. *Guyton and Hall's Textbook of Medical Physiology* (2000), the doctor's bible on physiology, indicates that most sugars or carbohydrates are converted to fat when consumed. Some of the glucose is converted to glycogen to be used for future energy needs. The body's ability to store or hold glycogen is limited to only a few hundred grams. The glucose that is not readily used or converted to glycogen is converted to fat, which is easily stored. The body can store many grams of fat (there are 2.2 pounds in each kilogram). This is not nutritional theory, but physiological fact. It is very easy to see the converted sugar as fat on us or on our friends!

Couple Guyton's facts on physiology with the additional facts from Wilson and Foster's *Textbook on Endocrinology,* 1992. Figure 1 of this book on page 33 makes the answers very apparent. They are simple, straightforward, and best yet, logical. The answers make good common sense, unlike the claims of most of today's diets. If we would not eat so much refined sugar and high-glycemic carbohydrates, the major portion of our population would not have these problems.

Unfortunately, American medical schools do not include much nutrition and dietetics in the curriculum. Please urge your doctor to read this book, critique it, check its conclusions with factual data in medical textbooks, and see if he or she does not arrive at a similar conclusion as that found in *Sugar Busters!*

Because high mean levels of insulin promote or accelerate obesity, hypertension, and heart disease, ask your doctor why so many nutritionists and even the American Diabetes Association still are recommending a carbohydrate-rich diet that causes our bodies to need more insulin.

The success stories have been exhilarating. There

is significant help available for both the borderline and full-fledged diabetic. We emphatically predict that, as more research is conducted, the general way of eating presented in this book, which is closer to the way our distant ancestors ate, will ultimately replace the current, faddish diets.

# 14 | Hypoglycemia

Hypoglycemia is a very common problem in our population. The term hypoglycemia is used to indicate a low blood sugar level, usually below 50 milligrams per deciliter (mg/dL) in adults. A blood sugar level below 40 mg/dL often requires medical attention. A person does not have to be a diabetic to have symptoms of hypoglycemia. Hypoglycemia frequently is the cause of the midday doldrums that many of us have experienced an hour or so after lunch. In the majority of instances, we have had a sugar-rich or high-glycemic, carbohydrate-rich meal that initially causes our blood sugar to rise with an associated significant insulin spike (Figure 1, page 18). But when the insulin does its work and the blood sugar begins to fall, it often drops to below normal. How far it falls below normal varies from individual to individual.

If you experience some of the symptoms discussed in this chapter, you may be prone to hypoglycemia, or you may just be unable to eat meals that are too full of high-glycemic-index foods. Research does point out that the more rapidly the blood sugar spikes and subsequently falls, the farther it will fall below normal (see Figure 7, page 64).

There are three categories of hypoglycemia: (1) reactive hypoglycemia, which we have discussed above and which is by far the most common form, (2) spontaneous, such as conditions caused by tumors of the pancreas; and (3) those that are induced by surgery involving the gastrointestinal tract.

The symptoms of hypoglycemia vary from lethargy to anxiety; for a small percentage of people, they even include depression. Mild to moderate symptoms include shakiness or trembling, pale skin, sweating, rapid pulse, hunger, irritability, poor coordination, dizziness, fatigue, sleepiness, headache, slurred speech, or daydreaming and lack of concentration.

Our first response often is to want to eat something, usually another high-glycemic carbohydrate that elevates our blood sugar, making us feel temporarily better. However, the consumption of any significant amount of a high-glycemic food will cause the spike-crash phenomenon to repeat itself, which will cause the urge for still more food. As a result, our blood sugar and insulin levels will fluctuate in a definitely unhealthy fashion that could have been avoided by eating properly in the first place. Just eat a piece of fruit or drink a little juice to give yourself a mild blood sugar rise so you will not experience the roller-coaster effect of high then low blood sugar that caused your hypoglycemia initially.

Diabetics, whether Type 1 or Type 2, often have bouts with hypoglycemia because insulin or oral diabetes medications, if not precisely balanced with proper amounts and timing of food consumption, can cause blood sugar to drop too low (hypoglycemia) as well as rise and remain too high (hyperglycemia).

Persons with significant symptoms of hypoglycemia should certainly consult their physician for competent professional advice. However, in the majority of cases, mild hypoglycemia is purely a result of eating a meal rich in high-glycemic carbohydrates. You frequently can avoid the symptoms associated with a low blood sugar level by following the *Sugar Busters!* lifestyle. And just think how much better your performance will be at work, at play, and even while driving after a low- rather than high-glycemic meal.

## 15 | Sugar Busters!
      for the Healthy Heart

Most of us follow a specific diet for one or two reasons, often to enhance our appearance or improve our cardiovascular health. Being slender seems to be considered more attractive by both men and women in America today. Most of us have tried to shed a few extra pounds before vacation or some important event. More recently, dieting to improve our health has been gaining greater importance. The cardiovascular system often is the target of these efforts. Therefore, we would like to elaborate a little about the cardiovascular system and the influence of diet.

Diseases of the cardiovascular system—primarily heart attack, hypertension, and stroke—are public enemy number one, accounting for twelve million deaths annually in the United States. Coronary heart disease is the leading cause of death in industrialized countries, and in the next ten years, coronary artery disease and stroke will become the leading cause of death in most developing countries.

Heart disease, stroke, and frequently hypertension are due to the deterioration of arteries through a process called atherosclerosis, arteriosclerosis, or just plain hardening of the arteries. This process is a natural phenomenon of aging. As we get older, so do our arteries. The smooth inner lining, called the intima, begins to crack when the elastic, muscular middle layer can no longer fully recoil after a pulse wave has expanded the vessel. In these cracks, platelets, fibrin, calcium, cholesterol, and fat accumulate, creating an atheroma, or plaque.

With continued stress on the arterial wall and further intimal (the innermost coat) disruption associated with blood flow turbulence, more material is deposited until the artery is narrowed significantly, producing reduced blood flow to the corresponding area of the body. We now refer to the process as a disease; its presence has caused a problem.

A frequent question asked of physicians is "How do I avoid getting arteriosclerosis?" The answer is easy: don't live long enough. Most patients do not like this alternative. However, some factors predispose us to premature or early arteriosclerosis and subsequently to cardiovascular disease. It is important to be aware of the risk factors and plan for them accordingly. Some we can alter. Others we cannot. But the knowledge gleaned from being aware of them usually is very helpful in assisting us to enhance cardiovascular fitness or health.

Initially, there were thought to be three major factors influencing early or premature development of arteriosclerosis: (1) elevated cholesterol, (2) elevated blood pressure, and (3) smoking. However, we now know that many other factors significantly influence the process as well. These include the following: heredity, diabetes, elevated triglycerides, obesity, stress, sugar, and sedentary lifestyle (Figure 12, below).

**Figure 12.**
## Arteriosclerotic cardiovascular disease risk factors.

| | |
|---|---|
| Heredity | Elevated triglycerides* |
| Smoking | Obesity* |
| High-blood pressure* | Stress* |
| Diabetes* | Sugar* |
| Elevated cholesterol* | Sedentary lifestyle* |

* Risk factors beneficially affected by the SUGAR BUSTERS! lifestyle.

Heredity, of all these factors, is the most important. Genetic factors contribute to an individual's susceptibility or resistance to cardiovascular disease. In addition, a part of the susceptibility and response to dietary factors is genetic in origin. Absolute control of the hereditary factor would involve picking our own parents, but for most of us, this is not an option! Those individuals with a strong family history of arteriosclerotic cardiovascular disease should be especially aware of the other risk factors so that they can alter their lifestyles to minimize the negative influence on their systems.

Smoking is a factor we all have the ability to control. The use of tobacco in all forms promotes the development of arteriosclerosis through a variety of mechanisms. The nicotine in tobacco is a powerful constrictor of blood vessels, causing reduced blood flow and a greater workload on the heart. Smokers have lower blood plasma levels of antioxidants, and we believe this makes them more susceptible to early plaque formation in arterial walls. The beneficial effects of many otherwise successful operations for complications of arteriosclerosis, such as coronary artery bypass, are more than cut in half by patients continuing to smoke.

Diabetes mellitus has long been associated with early, diffuse, and often prematurely fatal arteriosclerosis. However, the diabetics most severely affected are the 85 percent or so who are insulin-resistant. These individuals require increasingly higher plasma insulin levels to achieve the same result in regulating blood glucose. Elevated plasma insulin appears to promote fat deposits and smooth-muscle growth in arterial walls. Both of these processes are involved in plaque formation. In addition, high levels of insulin probably make it easier for the blood to coagulate, which obviously leads to easier clot formation and arterial blockage.

High blood pressure, or hypertension, is classified as "essential" in over 90 percent of instances. This means that we really do not know its cause, but we do know that it produces extra stress on both the heart and the arterial system. The diastolic, or bottom, pressure in the blood pressure reading is the force or resistance the heart and blood vessels are subjected to during the relaxation phase of the cardiac cycle, or heartbeat. The greater the stress during this phase, the more accelerated the aging, or deterioration of the arterial walls. This leads to loss of elastic tissue, cracking, and, as seen, plaque formation. Certainly, controlling blood pressure reduces stress on the cardiovascular system and promotes better long-term wear.

Hyperlipidemia (increased fat in the blood), especially hypercholesterolemia (elevated cholesterol), is associated with early onset of arteriosclerosis. Cholesterol is an important component in the formation of plaque. Cholesterol also is vital to the proper function of many bodily processes, such as steroid formation and the synthesis of lipoproteins (fat and protein combinations present in the blood), both of which are necessary for vital metabolic activities. Researchers also believe there is a link between cholesterol and insulin, as insulin-resistant diabetics, those with high plasma levels of insulin, have abnormally elevated cholesterol levels. The predominant cholesterol component in these individuals is the low-density lipoprotein (LDL) fraction, which frequently is referred to as "bad" cholesterol; remember, for LDL, *L* means lethal. Some components of cholesterol such as the high-density lipoprotein (HDL) fraction, especially HDL-2 and HDL-3, exert a protective effect on the cardio-vascular system; remember, for HDL, *H* means healthy.

Gender is a factor in the development of arteriosclerosis, and in this instance, women have an advantage at least until menopause. As seen in the next chapter, estrogen in premenopausal women decreases blood plasma insulin levels. This imparts a significant protective influence on the cardiovascular system against the development of arteriosclerosis. After menopause the incidence of arteriosclerosis in women begins to approach that seen in men.

Even in the absence of all risk factors, arteriosclerosis will occur; it is the natural aging process of our arteries. The theoretical maximum life expectancy of the cardiovascular system is approximately 120 years. There is a fine line between arteriosclerosis as an aging process and as a disease. In the elderly its presence often is termed normal aging, only to be reclassified as a disease when problems related to it arise. Rest assured, if we live long enough, we will develop arteriosclerosis, but consider the alternative!

Obesity has long been associated with early cardiovascular system problems. In age-adjusted populations where obesity is low, life expectancy is greater. Just compare France and the United States. Between the ages of sixteen and fifty, the French have 50 percent less obesity and 20 percent less cardiovascular and cholesterol problems than their U.S. counterparts. Excess body fat is deposited throughout all body tissues, and the cardiovascular system is no exception. The additional weight imposed by the extra pounds also creates an extra workload for the cardiovascular system. Exercise, although not mandatory for many people in achieving weight loss or stabilization, is a definite plus in terms of both cardiovascular benefits and overall health. A more complete discussion on this important component for an optimum lifestyle can be found in Chapter 17.

"We are what we eat" is an old adage familiar to almost everyone, but today this is becoming even more important as we better understand the full spectrum of nutrition and its effect on our various organ systems, especially the cardiovascular system.

Although fats and meats, especially red meats, have fallen into disfavor, and carbohydrates have been definitely "in," few people stopped to think about what happens to the excess sugar that is the end product of carbohydrate metabolism. Some sugar is used in our blood to maintain an adequate circulating blood glucose level, and some will replenish glycogen stores in the liver and muscles. But what happens to the rest? It is converted to fat.[1] Yes, most of our body fat comes from ingested sugar, not ingested fat. This conversion is facilitated by the hormone insulin.

In addition, insulin tends to block lipolysis, the

conversion of fat back to glucose. So, individuals with elevated insulin levels have a more difficult time burning fat for energy. Simply stated, they have a hard time losing weight!

Dietary sugar is now recognized as an independent risk factor for cardiovascular disease. This is caused by sugar's effect on insulin secretion. Insulin is now recognized as being atherogenic, that is, it causes the development of arteriosclerotic plaques in or on the walls of blood vessels. In addition, insulin is now known to cause cardiac enlargement, more specifically left ventricular hypertrophy. The left ventricle is the main pumping chamber of the heart and the chamber involved in 99 percent of heart attacks.

Insulin plays a very important role by influencing many of the other factors we have been discussing. An increased insulin level also promotes fat deposition and growth of smooth-muscle cells in the arteries (both necessary to plaque formation) and thus increases the tendency for clot formation. Two factors already discussed, estrogen and exercise, both decrease insulin resistance and are known to have a beneficial effect on the cardiovascular system in retarding the process of arteriosclerosis.

However, one group of individuals, regardless of how well they positively influence most of the significant risk factors, appear to develop an early, diffuse type of arteriosclerotic cardiovascular disease that often leads to premature heart attacks, stroke, and complications of hypertension. This group is comprised of insulin-resistant diabetics in whom the only primary measurable abnormality is elevated insulin levels. It has become readily apparent to us, as well as others, that insulin has many influences on the recognized processes responsible for the development of cardiovascular disease through arteriosclerosis. Therefore, the key to improving performance and health through nutrition involves insulin. Modulating insulin secretion through diet may just be the most important variable influencing the development of cardiovascular disease. Chapter 8 discusses how this modulation is accomplished, as well as how it affects weight gain or loss.

The *Sugar Busters!* lifestyle, by positively influencing eight of the ten major cardiovascular risk factors, helps you keep and maintain a "healthy heart." The *Sugar Busters!* way of eating will improve weight and insulin levels. This will promote better blood pressure and blood chemistry (cholesterol and triglycerides). Type 2 diabetes will either be entirely prevented or, at least better controlled. Many have noticed fewer mood swings and have had a reduction of stress. All of those factors will benefit cardiovascular health. Combat the number-one cause of premature death by following *Sugar Busters!* and greatly improve your risk profile for a healthy heart.

# 16 | Women and Weight Loss

Yes, women have more problems losing weight than men. However, some of the greatest *Sugar Busters!* successes have been among women. One lady we know was able to lose seventy-nine pounds over five months on the *Sugar Busters!* lifestyle.

Maggy Drezins Moity is a fifty-one-year-old from New Orleans who has had a weight problem all of her life until she started the *Sugar Busters!* lifestyle in 1997. When she graduated from high school, she weighed 120 pounds, but shortly after marriage and having children, her weight increased to 190 pounds. Following the sudden death of her husband, she began to eat excessively, finally reaching 319 pounds. Realizing something must be done, she reduced her food consumption and eliminated as much fat as she could from her diet. Over eighteen months she reduced her weight back to 190 pounds, where she again plateaued. Maggy was introduced to the *Sugar Busters!* lifestyle, and over the next five months she was able to lose seventy-nine pounds, dropping to her current weight of 111 pounds. She says that *Sugar Busters!* is the most fantastic diet ever. She has always been a sweets freak, yet this way of eating has taken away her craving for sweets. Her energy, performance, and sense of well-being are all better. To help keep herself on track, Maggy makes a point of reviewing *Sugar Busters!* every month and even refers to the book as "my bible." Following the *Sugar Busters!* lifestyle has created a new figure and a new life for Maggy, who has married again. Maggy says, "I think *Sugar Busters!* is great!"

We have just recontacted Maggy, who has now been on the *Sugar Busters!* lifestyle for five years. Maggy is still 200 pounds down in her weight and says she is full of energy and feels great! Yet all the prominent expert-critics continue to say that diets that contain more than the historically recommended amount of protein (around 15 percent of the diet) only cause a temporary loss of water and weight. Please explain how Ms. Moity could have been carrying 200 pounds of water rather than fat on her body. And do they consider five years a temporary weight loss? This is not a testimonial from a "Joe" or "Sally" or "Jim" or "Jane." Maggy, as with all our testimonials, is a real person.

Maggy also commented on the total volume of food she has been consuming. She says she is continuing to eat larger volumes of food, albeit different (lower-glycemic) food, than she was eating when she weighed 319 pounds or when she had plateaued at her pre-*Sugar Busters!* weight of 190 pounds.

We salute you, Maggy Moity, for helping to enlighten all the outdated experts who cannot seem to understand some very straightforward physiological processes regarding nutrition and metabolism.

Another lady, Lala Ball Cooper, from Memphis, Tennessee, wrote the following about her experience with *Sugar Busters!* "My *Sugar Busters!* journey began eighteen months ago. How I found the motivation even to begin the trip is still a conundrum. I had, after all, long before that particular spring, completely abandoned any hope of unloading any portion of my substantial cushion of padding that surrounded what really was in fact a medium frame. A literal lifetime of weight battling stretched behind me as far as my memory could track—to early elementary school at least. Forever in search of a solution, and perennially unsuccessful in finding one, I had tried every year's dieting fad one right after the other until I had finally arrived at the point where the news of a possible new solution—even one accompanied by the glitziest media promo—could no longer pique my interest. I can't, then, explain how I found the motivation even to investigate the *Sugar Busters!* book. I am still amazed that I bought a copy and even more amazed that I read it and tried it in the first place, so high was the level of skepticism at the time and so low the level of hope that any plan would ever succeed for me.

"*Sugar Busters!* began to work immediately. Pounds started to fall away swiftly, but I was so heavy when I began that no one noticed at the high school where I teach, even after two months. I told no one that I was dieting (we perpetually fat folks finally learn not to advertise after so many failures). With my secret still intact, I spent the summer continuing to lose steadily. After I returned to teaching in the fall with a noticeably smaller body, my secret was out.

"I am now 124 pounds lighter than when I began. Although I lost the bulk of my weight during the first eight months, I still continue to lose, although much more slowly now. The best part of all is that I haven't gained any weight back. To accomplish this I've approached my new success with a new attitude. I know that *Sugar Busters!* for me is not something that I will have the luxury of discarding after I reach my desirable weight. It is going to have to remain a habit of life if I intend to keep my weight off. Because it is based on valid nutritional principles and has eliminated the big enemy of dieters, deprivation, continuing this plan is something that I feel that I can reasonably expect to do over the long haul. I am healthier than I have ever been, as attested to by the blood chemistry reports I get from my doctor when I go for annual checkups. For the first time ever I really believe that I am going to be able to put a heavy-weight history be-hind me."

## Congratulations Lala Ball Cooper!

However, some women on *Sugar Busters!* have become frustrated because of experiencing slower results in weight loss than their male counterparts. Michel Montignac's most recent book, *La Méthode Montignac Spéciale Femme,* addresses this problem.

Montignac identifies four points that he feels make it more difficult for women to lose weight. These are: (1) women are more sedentary than men; (2) women snack more than men; (3) women diet more than men, so their bodies are more resistant to diets; and (4) women frequently are on hormone supplementation, which makes it more difficult to lose weight and actually may cause them to gain weight. Although the authors of *Sugar Busters!* are not in total agreement with Montignac, we do feel there is merit to some of his points.

In general, women may exercise less vigorously and have less muscle mass to burn energy sources than their male counterparts do. More men jog or use highly resistant exercise machines, while women tend to participate more in aerobic exercise programs. However, you must remember that thou-sands of people are losing weight by closely follow-ing the *Sugar Busters!* way of eating even in the absence of exercise.

Women who do not work outside the home tend to snack more than either working women or their male counterparts. This is only natural because someone frequently in and out of the kitchen has more opportunity to eat than someone who is away from home most of the day.

Women taking certain hormone supplements, such as birth control pills, can have significant problems losing weight, especially if progesterone is involved. Progesterone increases appetite and definitely promotes fat storage. Many gynecologists use progesterone as an appetite stimulant in patients recovering from surgery or other procedures where improved nutrition and weight gain are desirable. If a woman is on hormonal supplementation of any kind, she should not discontinue it on her own but should seek medical consultation.

Many menopausal and postmenopausal women have been placed on hormone therapy combining estrogen and progesterone, which has made it more difficult for these women to lose weight. Based on a study of 16,000 women without heart disease, the government has recently circulated warnings that this combination has been proven to increase the relative risk of a woman developing heart disease by 29 percent, strokes by 41 percent, invasive breast cancer by 26 percent, blood clots in the veins by 107 percent, and blood clots in the lungs by 113 percent. While the discontinuation of this therapy may be bad news for women with hot flashes and other symptoms, it will be good news for those women who have been having trouble losing weight.

Estrogen alone, however, may be beneficial to women trying to lose weight because it increases insulin sensitivity. Estrogen, therefore, acts similarly to exercise as an adjunct to the *Sugar Busters!* lifestyle. All these things assist in lowering insulin levels.

Moreover, women, on the average, are genetically more efficient at fat storage than men. This difference begins at birth and continues throughout life. Because women must support both themselves and the developing fetus during pregnancy, and both themselves and the nursing infant during lactation, their systems are more efficient at storing reserves that are available to support them during these times.

The problem many women have in losing weight is real, and they need to review carefully all of the points above in trying to achieve the best results from the *Sugar Busters!* lifestyle. Obviously, some factors, such as hormones, are a stronger influence than others. However, for many women, it is important not to dismiss any of the points. For them, strict attention to detail will ultimately yield the satisfactory results that we are continuing to see in most women on the *Sugar Busters!* lifestyle.

According to Dr. Christiane Northrup in *The*

*Wisdom of Menopause,* about 25 percent of women have thyroid problems by the time they reach peri-menopause. Since low thyroid function can cause your metabolic rate to drop, you should have your thyroid checked if you are adhering to the *Sugar Busters!* lifestyle but are not seeing results.

Another significant benefit of following the *Sugar Busters!* lifestyle was pointed out by Dr. Bennie R. Nobles of New Orleans. It was recently found that a common cause of fertility problems in female patients, specifically polycystic ovarian syndrome, was related to increased insulin resistance, which is common in obese women. Those patients, in an attempt to keep their blood sugar normal, would produce an abnormal amount of insulin to keep from becoming diabetic. After being treated with Glucophage, a drug that is known to lower insulin requirements, many women began ovulating and became pregnant. It has now been found that many of the same benefits can be achieved by having the women follow a low-glycemic diet accompanied by exercise. The *Sugar Busters!* lifestyle, which lowers average blood insulin levels, has been effective in helping some of these women lower their previously elevated insulin levels and has helped some of them become pregnant. We thank Dr. Nobles for relating this additional benefit of the *Sugar Busters!* lifestyle.

Interestingly, many women on *Sugar Busters!* who have also been on hormones have commented that, in spite of achieving only minimal success in losing weight, their dress size has decreased significantly, indicating that a redistribution of weight is occurring. This has led to a greater sense of well-being and improved self-image. Being lean and fit is a fantastic feeling. Do not deny yourself this attainable pleasure!

# 17 | Exercise

Just over a hundred years ago, exercise was difficult to avoid. There were no automobiles, airplanes, subways, or electrical appliances, all of which have now taken "movement" out of our daily lives. Today, our world encourages us to be lazy and expend few calories. Our heart rate, muscle tone, and insulin sensitivity deteriorate, and our fat storage and disease rates go up.

A sedentary lifestyle definitely does not have a positive influence on the cardiovascular system or allow us to achieve optimum health. Inactivity may not be significantly harmful, but reasonable exercise is beneficial. Exercise decreases blood pressure, decreases serum lipoproteins (especially the bad cholesterol components), decreases obesity, decreases insulin resistance by increasing insulin sensitivity, decreases basal insulin levels, reduces the tendency for blood clot formation, and stimulates the breakdown of clots that have already been produced. However, the most common problem with exercise programs is that most people's intentions exceed their actual performance. At the other extreme, some people spend so much time and effort on high-impact exercises, like running marathons, that many end up with spinal or other joint problems.

The maximum cardiovascular benefit can be achieved by exercising on a regular basis, four times a week, so that you elevate your resting heart rate to a prescribed level for a period of twenty consecutive minutes. To determine your ideal heart rate during exercise, you should subtract your age from 220 and multiply this number by 0.70, or 70 percent. This is the heart rate you should sustain for twenty minutes during an exercise program four times a week. If you choose to exercise more frequently and/or for longer periods of time, that is your prerogative, but from a cardiovascular standpoint, exercising to elevate your heart rate to the prescribed level four times a week achieves the maximum benefit from exercise. A word of caution: if you are over fifty years of age, have cardiac risk factors, or are not accustomed to exercising, consult your physician before beginning your exercise program.

Exercise is a tremendous adjunct to the *Sugar Busters!* lifestyle. Both help us lower our mean insulin levels, and that is the goal we are all trying to achieve for healthier and longer lives. Exercise positively influences many of the risk factors governing our overall fitness as well as the fitness of our cardiovascular systems.

While this chapter is quite short, it is intended to give you a simple formula that will allow you to derive significant benefit from whatever form of exercise you choose. There must be thousands of machines on which you can exercise plus millions of miles of trails, roads, and sidewalks on which to jog or walk. Just get your heart rate up to the prescribed number, hold it there for at least twenty minutes, do it several days a week, and you will have done what it takes to reap many of the benefits of an exercise program.

Exercise alone will not always cause weight loss or even weight stabilization. This is true even for some people who exercise very strenuously. Often, a proper diet must accompany the program. Consider the letter we received from Anne Morley of Houston, Texas, that addresses exactly this point.

"I wanted to let you know how wonderfully successful I have been with your *Sugar Busters!* program.

"I have taught aerobics for eighteen years and my body had gotten used to the workout. I am about to turn forty and my metabolism went from the efficiency of a Porsche to that of a VW Bug. Your program was the only thing that has worked for me. I have lost over twenty pounds and feel great. I have a ton of energy. I currently teach power cycling and tae bo classes fifteen hours per week.

"The other wonderful side benefit from your *Sugar Busters!* lifestyle is that my children are much less hyper in the evenings. I can see a huge difference in my preteen daughter and, also, some of her friends. We are all trying to steer ourselves from becoming victims of 'technological obesity' (too much TV, too much time on the computer).

"Many of my aerobic students have incorporated your program in their lives and are thoroughly enjoying it. I am a firm believer in *Sugar Busters!* and am trying to spread the word." Thank you, Anne, for providing the proof that exercise alone does not always accomplish weight control or weight loss.

Regular exercise usually increases bone density. If your doctor has informed you that you exhibit any of the signs of having osteoporosis, or if you are in a high-risk group, such as postmenopausal women with small bones, you would be wise to add some weight-bearing exercise to help keep your bones strong. These resistance-type exercises should be done at least twice a week and for twenty to thirty minutes per session.

Since exercise increases insulin sensitivity, it is also very important in the treatment of, as well as in helping prevent the development of diabetes.

If the above reasons are not enough to get you moving several times a week, consider the following. Stanford University and Veterans Affairs Health Care Systems researchers studied more than 6,000 middle-aged men for thirteen years and found that the men who had the best exercise capacity clearly outlived those with a lower exercise capacity. Those with the lowest exercise capacity had more than four times the risk of premature death than those with the highest capacity. Exercise capacity turned out to be a better predictor of death than even heart disease, diabetes, high blood pressure, or smoking.[1] Get moving!

# 18 | Super Foods

All of the foods described in this section are included in the very extensive list of acceptable foods for the *Sugar Busters!* lifestyle. We feel, however, that those found below do have special merit for anyone who is on any kind of balanced diet. These foods are loaded with vitamins, minerals, and in most cases fiber, so they pack an impressive nutritional punch as well as delivering strong preventive medicine.

With only one exception, some of the beans, our distant ancestors ate these foods raw. We still eat many of them raw, and there are healthy people around the world that do eat all but the beans raw. Fortunately, with proper preparation and cooking, most foods can retain their super nutritive punch and be delicious as well.

To assist you in consuming these foods in the most enjoyable manner, we have included some very basic recipes when appropriate, at the end of this chapter. The foods are not listed in any particular order because we strongly urge you to partake of all these foods, which can help ensure consumption of the vitamins, minerals, and fiber you require for optimum health. You also have the opportunity to enjoy eating these foods instead of going to the trouble and expense of taking many of the supplements that are so aggressively marketed to you today. Regulation on the claims made by many pill and potion pushers are very weak on nonprescription products, and some products have even been recalled after they products have been determined to be toxic to humans after prolonged use.

Feeding your body with these super foods presents your digestive system with the opportunity to extract the benefits your body requires in exactly the manner for which your digestive system was designed by Mother Nature. As mentioned in Chapter 5, researchers continue to isolate important new substances in the three food groups, and many of these important substances can't be found in any of today's pills or potions. Consider too that the various nutrients in wholesome fresh foods may work together in ways that we don't yet fully understand—and that it's impossible to duplicate these complex combinations in a pill.

Please notice something else about these super foods. All but the seafood, olive oil, lean meats, and portions of the milk are carbohydrates and thus are converted into glucose (sugar) in our bodies to produce the energy we require. All but sweet potatoes are low-glycemic carbs, and sweet potatoes are only in the moderate range. Well, so much for *Sugar Busters!* being a low-carbohydrate diet! We have always said *Sugar Busters!* is simply about eating the right (low-glycemic, high-fiber) carbohydrates.

Another good thing to remember each day is that to eat right, eat something bright. Red, orange, yellow, or dark green fruits and vegetables generally have more vitamins, minerals, and other nutrients than the less colorful foods.

If you do not like the taste of some of these foods, find a way to disguise them. Your poor ancestors, who probably ate every edible thing they could get their hands on, did not have the arsenal of seasonings and spices you have at your fingertips. They had no A1 Sauce, refined sugar, garlic, or salt. As you eat your next meal, think about your ancestors, tip your hat to them, and enjoy the pleasures of modern eating (except for those high-glycemic carbs)!

## 1. Greens—Kale, Collards, and Spinach

The creator of Popeye must have peeked at the nutrition table when he chose spinach as the food that made Popeye so strong. (He even chose "Olive Oyl," also on our list, as Popeye's companion.) We should all thank him for recommending such a nutritious food in a way that stimulated its consumption by many of us who otherwise would not have eaten spinach. Popeye was very fortunate, however, that Bluto (who got fat eating his hamburgers on white bread) did not dine on kale and collards because their nutritive value can even exceed that of spinach in some categories.

That said, whether you choose Popeye's spinach or the greens of "King Kale" or the "Collard Queen," you have chosen a super food. These greens and others, to a lesser degree, contain vitamin A, carotenoids, and vitamin C, all powerful antioxidants. They also contain a lot of calcium and fiber. All are extremely low-glycemic and can be eaten in large quantities.

Nutritional research on macular degeneration has shown that consumption of lutein and zeaxanthin, but not beta-carotene, is associated with a reduced risk for macular degeneration. People who ate the most lutein and zeaxanthin had a 57 percent lower risk for macular degeneration than people who ate the least. The three top sources of lutein are kale, collard greens, and spinach.[1] Any of these greens can be found fresh, frozen, or in cans in the grocery.

## 2. Sweet Potatoes

What a great substitute for the high-glycemic white potato, which contains much less nutritive value and less fiber. Sweet potatoes contain abundant carotenoids and are also high in vitamins C and E, potassium, and fiber. Sweet potatoes can also satisfy many people's sweet tooth. Some tribes today (i.e. in Irian Jaya) eat a type of sweet potato almost exclusively and are in apparent good health.

## 3. Fruit—Cantaloupe, Blueberries, Oranges, and Tomatoes

Cantaloupe is very high in carotenoids, with one cup delivering the entire recommended daily allowance of vitamins A and C. Blueberries have been shown in recent studies to be high in bioflavonoids and thus a good antioxidant and blood thinner that helps fight cardiovascular diseases. Oranges are high in vitamin C, folic acid, and fiber and make a very good and easily transportable snack. Tomatoes are high in vitamin A and have been indicated in many recent studies to lower the risk of prostate cancer. Also, according to research on nearly 10,000 people in the National Health and Nutrition Examination Survey Epidemiological Follow-up Study, people who ate three or more fruits and vegetables a day had 27 percent fewer strokes, were 42 percent less likely to die from a stroke, and were 25 percent less likely to die from heart disease.[2]

## 4. Green Vegetables—Broccoli

Broccoli is easily found and inexpensive. It is high in vitamins A and C, calcium and potassium, and folic acid. Broccoli can be eaten raw, steamed, or cooked with other vegetables or cheese dishes.

## 5. Beans, Lentils

Beans and lentils are not only good for you but are the least expensive substitute for white potatoes, white rice, and corn. They are high in soluble fiber, iron, potassium, calcium, and magnesium, and very high in folic acid. Researchers from Tulane University and the National Heart, Lung, and Blood Institute followed the eating patterns of 9,600 people for nineteen years and found that those who ate legumes (beans, peas, and peanuts) only one time a week were 22 percent more likely to develop heart disease than those who ate legumes at least four times a week.[3]

## 6. Nuts—Almonds, Walnuts

Almonds and walnuts are high in fiber, vegetable protein, vitamin E, and the good kinds of fat. Almonds are very rich in calcium and walnuts are rich in vitamin $B_6$ and alpha-linolenic acid, an omega-3 fatty acid. Walnuts are also high in the heart-healthy omega-3 fatty acids. Nurses who ate nuts five times a week versus once a week had 20 percent less diabetes.[4] They make excellent snacks or substitutes for desserts and are among the easiest of all foods to transport.

### 7. Whole Grains—Wheat, Oats, and Barley

Whole-grain wheat products are high in fiber, the B vitamins, and vitamin E. Whole-grain breads contain many more natural vitamins and nutrients than the few vitamins added back to the enriched breads and white flours. Whole oats, barley, and rye are also good foods, with oats containing an impressive amount of soluble fiber, which has been shown to help lower LDL (the "bad" cholesterol).

### 8. Seafood—Salmon, Tuna, Mackerel, and Sardines

These cold-water fish are very high in the good omega-3 fatty acids, which have been shown to have beneficial effects in reducing cardiovascular disease. In the Physicians Health Study that followed 22,000 initially healthy men for seventeen years, the men with the highest blood levels of omega-3 fatty acids had an 80 percent lower chance of dying suddenly from a cardiovascular-related event compared to the men with the lowest levels.[5] Salmon, more easily catchable than the others, must have been a staple for our ancestors who, over the last one million years, found our earth gripped by ice ages 90 percent of the time.

## 9. Oils—Olive Oil

Olive oil is primarily a monosaturated fat (the good fat) and has been a staple in countries that have exhibited a much lower incidence of cardiovascular disease than those following a modern Western diet. Olive oil is a good source of the not-so-easily-found vitamin E.

## 10. Proteins—Liver and Lean Meats

While many lean meats deliver abundant proteins that our bodies need as the building blocks for cell growth and assimilation of many vitamins and minerals, liver stands out in its abundance of vitamins A, C, $B_2$, $B_{12}$, and iron. Liver is also surprisingly low in saturated fat when compared to other red meats. Of course, most fish and fowl are low in saturated fat and are also excellent sources of protein.

## 11. Milk

Milk was not a staple for our ancestors. However, the foods listed above, as well as other acceptable foods not discussed here, generally do not supply the full amount of calcium our bodies require in an era where three-quarters of Americans do not exercise (exercise increases the density and strength of our bones) and many others, particularly those in the higher latitudes, do not get enough sun to help their bodies make vitamin D (vitamin D is necessary for the absorption of calcium). To get enough calcium, we recommend consumption of either milk (skim is okay) or cheese in the diet to ensure that we are getting reasonable amounts of calcium. If you are lactose-intolerant (unable to digest lactose, the sugar found in milk), you should get your calcium elsewhere, however.

## Honorable Mention

### Flaxseeds

These small seeds are full of omega-3 fatty acids, fiber, protein, and phytoestrogens. The omega-3 alpha-linoleic acid has been shown to reduce blood clotting, and the phytoestrogen lignan is thought to help prevent hormone-related cancers (such as breast cancer and prostate cancer) and raise the HDL "good" cholesterol. The most effective way to consume flaxseed is to eat them freshly ground, or to remember to chew them very well, as they can pass undigested if left whole. Flaxseeds can be added to cereals quite easily.

### Chocolate

Find yourself some high-cocoa (>60 percent), low-sugar chocolate and you will be consuming high amounts of polyphenols and other flavonoids that are strong antioxidants. A study reported in the

*American Journal of Clinical Nutrition* in November 2001 found that a diet supplemented with cocoa powder and dark chocolate slowed the oxidation of LDL ("bad" cholesterol) and increased the level of HDL ("good" cholesterol).[6]

While you can get all the health and nutrition benefits from the basic recipes included on the following pages, feel free to add whatever herbs, spices or seasonings you would like to add to enhance their flavor for your own palate.

## Lentils

1 lb. dried lentils
6–8 cups of water
1 piece smoked ham hock, 4 slices of bacon, or
   ½ lb. sliced sausage
Salt to taste

Sort and wash beans. Add beans and meat and salt to pot with water. Bring to a boil, cover, reduce heat, and simmer for 45 minutes or until lentils are tender or al dente.

Eliminate meat if you prefer just beans. Garlic salt can be substituted if desired.

*Serves 6*

### Steamed Broccoli

2 large stalks of broccoli, washed and separated into
    florets
1 cup water
Salt to taste

Bring water and salt to a slow simmer in a medium
saucepan. Add broccoli and cook several minutes
until tender.

*Serves 4*


### Balsamic Broccoli

½ cup water
1 teaspoon salt
3 large stalks broccoli, cut into 1-inch florets
1 tablespoon olive oil
4 cloves garlic, peeled and crushed
1 small jalapeño pepper, cored, seeded, deveined,
    and minced
¼ cup balsamic vinegar

Bring the water to a boil in a 3-quart saucepan.
    Add the salt and broccoli. Bring back to a boil
and boil until the broccoli is crisp-tender, about
3 minutes. Drain and set aside. Meanwhile, combine the oil, garlic, and jalapeño pepper in a
medium skillet over medium heat. Sauté until

the garlic has just begun to brown, 1 to 2 minutes. Add the broccoli and vinegar, reduce the heat to medium-low, and cook for two minutes.

*Serves 4*

### Broccoli Au Gratin

2 large stalks of broccoli, washed and separated into
  florets
1 cup water
1 cup shredded cheddar cheese
1 medium onion, diced
Salt and pepper to taste

Steam broccoli as in previous recipe, but only cook until slightly soft. Drain and place in a baking dish with onions. Sprinkle with the cheese, salt, and pepper. Bake at 325° for 20 minutes or until onions are soft and clear and cheese is well melted.

*Serves 4 to 6*

### Boiled Kale and/or Collard Greens

2 quarts water
2 bunches kale and/or collard greens, stems
  removed and washed
1 small ham hock, optional
Salt and pepper to taste

Bring water to a boil and add the greens and ham hock, salt, and pepper. Cook until tender. Drain and serve as is or sprinkle with vinegar from a bottle of peppers and vinegar.

*Serves 4*

### Skillet-Grilled Salmon

Four 6-ounce fresh salmon fillets
½ teaspoon garlic salt
1 large lemon, halved
2 tablespoons olive oil
2 tablespoons chopped fresh flat-leaf parsley

Sprinkle the fillets with garlic salt. Squeeze lemon juice generously over the fish. Pour the oil into the bottom of a large skillet and preheat over high heat. Add the fillets, and sprinkle with half of the parsley. Cook until the fish is browned on the bottom, about 2 minutes. Turn, sprinkle with the rest of the parsley, and cook for about 2 minutes more, until browned on the second side.

Serve immediately.

*Serves 4*

## *Creole Spinach*

Two 10-ounce packages chopped frozen spinach
¾ stick butter
1 medium yellow onion, chopped
2 cloves garlic, chopped
Salt and ground black pepper to taste
3 tablespoons stone-ground whole-wheat flour
1⅓ cups low-fat milk
2 cups coarsely grated Velveeta cheese

Preheat the oven to 325 degrees. Cook the spinach according to package directions, drain, and squeeze out excess water. Melt the butter in a medium skillet over medium heat. Add the onion, garlic, salt, and pepper. Stirring constantly, cook until the onion softens a bit, about 3 minutes, and then add the spinach. In a small bowl, dissolve the flour in the milk. Add to the skillet. Stir in the cheese. Scrape into a 1-quart ovenproof casserole dish and bake until lightly browned on top, about 25 minutes.

*Serves 6 to 8*

## *Sautéed Spinach*

2 strips bacon
2 tablespoons olive oil
1 pound fresh sliced white button mushrooms or

one 4-ounce can sliced mushrooms, rinsed and drained
One 10-ounce package fresh salad spinach, rinsed, drained, and torn
2 green onions, chopped (including some of the green tops)
Salt and ground black pepper to taste

In a large skillet over medium-low heat, cook the bacon until crisp, 6 to 8 minutes. Remove the bacon to paper towels to drain, leaving the drippings in the pan. Add the oil to the bacon drippings. Add the mushrooms and sauté over medium-high heat until tender, about 3 minutes. Add the spinach and green onions; reduce the heat to medium-low and cook, stirring constantly, until wilted, 3 to 4 minutes. Season with salt and pepper. Crumble the bacon into the spinach and serve while still warm.

*Serves 3 to 4*

### Baked Sweet Potato

1 sweet potato, about 6 oz.
2 pats butter
Salt and pepper to taste

Wrap potato in a paper towel and microwave for 3 to 5 minutes until somewhat soft to the squeeze. Slice open and serve with butter, salt, and pepper.

*Serves 1*

### Mashed Sweet Potatos

3 sweet potatoes, 6–8 oz. each
1 teaspoon cinnamon
½ teaspoon black pepper
Salt to taste

Wrap potatoes in paper towels and cook in microwave 10 to 15 minutes until soft to the squeeze. Remove skin and mash. Add cinnamon, pepper, and salt and mix well.

*Serves 4 to 6*

### Sautéed Sweet Potatoes

2 sweet potatoes, about 6 oz. each, cut into
   ¼-inch slices
2 tablespoons olive oil
Salt and/or other spices to taste

Warm oil in large skillet over medium heat. Add sliced potatoes and cook, turning once, until potatoes are soft to the prongs of a fork. Sprinkle with salt and/or other spices and serve.

*Serves 4 to 6*

### Tomatoes Stuffed with Spinach

Four 10-ounce packages frozen whole-leaf spinach
8 medium tomatoes
One 8-ounce jar Jalapeño Cheez Whiz
1 teaspoon onion powder
¾ teaspoon garlic powder
⅛ teaspoon salt
1 teaspoon ground black pepper
8 pats butter

Preheat the oven to 350 degrees. Cook the spinach according to package directions. Meanwhile, slice 1 inch off the top of each tomato. With a spoon, scoop out the inside pulp, taking care to remove the seeds and leaving the meat attached to the outer skin intact. Squeeze excess water from the spinach and put it in a large bowl. Stir in the Cheez Whiz. Add the onion powder, garlic powder, salt, and pepper. Mix well. Divide the mixture among the tomato shells. Top each with a pat of butter. Place the stuffed tomatoes in a baking dish and add just enough water to cover the bottom. Bake for about 10 minutes.

*Serves 8*

## *Fresh Spinach Salad with Bacon*

One 10-ounce package fresh salad spinach
3 strips crisp cooked bacon, crumbled
One 4-ounce can hearts of palm, drained and sliced
1 teaspoon garlic salt
Scant ½ cup Cider Vinaigrette (recipe below)
2 hard-boiled eggs, sliced

In a large bowl, mix together the spinach, bacon, hearts of palm, and garlic salt. Add the Cider Vinaigrette, toss to coat, and garnish with the sliced egg.

*Serves 4*

## *Cider Vinaigrette*

¼ cup olive oil
Juice of ½ lemon
1 tablespoon apple cider vinegar
1 clove garlic, mashed
¼ teaspoon Lawry's or other seasoned salt
⅛ teaspoon ground black pepper

In a small bowl, whisk together the oil, lemon juice, vinegar, garlic, seasoned salt, and pepper.

*Makes about 1 cup.*

**Note:** This is good on almost any type of green salad.

### Grilled Cherry Tomatoes

1 carton small or cherry tomatoes, sliced in half
2 tablespoons minced garlic
2 tablespoons olive oil
1 tablespoon thyme
2 tablespoons Parmesan cheese

Place sliced tomatoes on broiler pan. Sprinkle with garlic, thyme, olive oil, and Parmesan and grill in oven at 325° for 5 minutes or until slightly browned.

*Serves 8*


### Black, Red, or Pinto Beans

1 lb. dried black, red, or pinto beans
1 ham hock, 4 slices bacon, or ½ lb. sliced Kielbasa sausage (optional)
1 yellow onion, diced
1 teaspoon garlic salt
1 tablespoon chili powder (optional)
Salt to taste

Sort and wash beans. Place in pot with 8 cups of water, bring to a boil, and boil for 10 minutes. Remove from heat, cover, and let soak for 1 hour. Drain and place in pot with 6 cups water (8 cups water if you want beans more like a soup) and add ham hock, if desired, onion, garlic salt, and chili powder if desired. Cook at a low boil, partially covered 1½ to 2 hours. Taste after 1 hour and add additional salt if required. Serve in a bowl or on a plate.

*Serves 6 to 8*

Note: For navy or white beans, use the same recipe as above, except we do not recommend using the optional chili powder.

# 19 | Soft Drinks, Hard Facts

The single leading source of added sugars in the average American's diet comes from the consumption of soft drinks. On average, we each consume over 55 gallons of soft drinks a year.[1] The U.S. Department of Agriculture reports that half of all Americans drink sodas daily, and most sodas consumed are not the diet type. At 10 teaspoons of sugar in each 12-ounce can of soda (rounded down for diet soda consumption), the rough math yields about 40 pounds of sugar per person per year, or about 30 percent of the total added sugar consumed per person each year. Many young people consume much more.

The British medical journal *The Lancet* reported on a recent U.S. study of 548 ethnically diverse children ages seven to eleven that concluded that the consumption of sugar-sweetened drinks and childhood obesity are definitely linked.[2] For each additional such drink, the children had a 60 percent greater chance of becoming obese! Unfortunately, sodas, with their nutritionless calories, are being consumed in copious quantities by our children.

The USDA report indicates that two-thirds of female children and three-fourths of male children drink sodas daily.

Further, soft drinks are replacing nutritious or neutral drinks such as water, fruit juices, and milk. In the USDA Nationwide Food Consumption Survey, conducted between 1977–78 and 1994–95, milk consumption in men decreased 17 percent and soft drink consumption increased 162 percent!

Furthermore, phosphoric acid, which is present in most soft drinks, can interfere with the efficient absorption of calcium.[3] It is easy to see why our children are not developing the proper bone density early in life and so will be much more likely to have osteoporotic problems, including bone fractures, later on.[4] The fact that the sodas are replacing the consumption of calcium-rich milk or fruit juices amplifies the problem. High phosphoric acid intake together with low calcium intake can alter the calcium-phosphorus ratio and decrease calcium absorption. Also, calcium cannot be absorbed when vitamin D is deficient, and since our children are spending less time outdoors, where the sun promotes vitamin D production in our bodies, this replacement of sodas for milk becomes even more of a problem.

During the meteoric rise in adult and childhood obesity and diabetes in the last thirty-five years, the consumption of sodas has roughly tripled. Chapters 5, 6, and 8 tell you of the other problems brought on by obesity and diabetes. Many parents and their teenagers start their day with a sugar-loaded, caffeine-rich, but "nutritionless" cola. Not only are they missing the vitamins and minerals they would get with a breakfast containing whole-grain products and fruit or eggs, but also, as mentioned above, they are even depleting their bodies of calcium.

Snacks from vending machines, many of which contain high-glycemic sugars and refined flours, are often consumed with a sugar-filled soft drink. Even when the snack is relatively low on the glycemic scale—nuts, for instance—the soda raises the body's insulin response, and the body's cells are signaled to store whatever fat may be circulating in the system, regardless of its origin.

To put 10 teaspoons of added sugar per regular soft drink into perspective, how many of you would scoop 10 teaspoons of sugar into a glass of tea and then sit and drink it? Nobody would, but the soft drinks are designed in such a way that neither the sugar nor the sodium or any other ingredients overpower your taste buds.

Are colas and other caffeine-containing soft drinks addictive? The John Hopkins University Hospital and many other authorities say caffeine is addictive. Each cola contains about one-half as much caffeine, 45 milligrams, as a cup of instant coffee, and somewhat more caffeine than an 8-ounce glass of, say, iced tea. If these colas are being consumed routinely—especially with chocolate candy, which also contains caffeine—it is easy to see that our children's bodies can get "wired" on caffeine. This can cause nervousness, anxiety, and sleeplessness. Caffeine is like a lot of other compounds in that your body can tolerate small or moderate amounts without ill effects, but too much can cause problems.

What can you as an individual or parent do about the epidemic overindulgence in these soft drinks that hit your waistline and health so hard? First, get them out of the household pantry. If they are not there to drink, they cannot be drunk by yourself or the members of your family. Replace the soft drinks with decaffeinated coffees or teas (green tea tastes pleasant, is full of antioxidants, and doesn't suppress your hunger for other nutritious foods). Most whole fruits contain large quantities of water and make a much better snack than any of the sodas. No-sugar-added lemonade is also good for you. Some of the no-sugar-added sports drinks, such as Refresher, which is full of electrolytes, which are needed after exercise, are much better choices.

Second, let's take the lead from others who have taken positive action to have soft drinks eliminated from the schools, where they are so handy to our children all day. California has prohibited soft drinks from elementary and middle schools during certain hours. Several school districts in Texas have done likewise.

There is a drive under way in Wyoming, led by

the former head of the state's dental association, Dr. Jim Landers, a medical doctor, and a leading nutritionist, to ban soft drink vending machines altogether for grades K through 12.[5] They have encountered strong opposition from the soft drink industry, as well as some of the schools themselves, which make considerable income from the sales of these beverages, and this has slowed their progress. The group is still hopeful that the voters will see the higher wisdom of putting the present and future health of the children ahead of a few dollars for the school system.

The Wyoming group points out that the consumption of soft drinks is causing a rise in tooth decay, weak bones, obesity, and diabetes and that 80 percent of overweight children will become fat adults. Looked at properly, the cost savings from prevention of the many health problems for our overall society will far more than offset our current loss of revenue for our schools.

Groups in other states such as Minnesota, Ohio, and North Carolina also are attempting to restrict the free flow of sodas to our children. We believe people are justified in trying to eliminate empty-calorie, harmful products from the schools, where children are developing their nutrition habits.

# 20 | Reading Labels

The two biggest minefields we have in trying to read food labels are deciphering the total added sugar content in grams relative to the naturally occurring sugars and trying to figure out whether a product is really "whole-wheat," "whole-grain" or "stone (coarsely)-ground," or whether it contains only a splash of any of the three.

Whole-grain products are great. Whole-grain wheat products have a lot of fiber, vitamin E, B-6, magnesium, zinc, potassium, copper, and hundreds of phytochemicals that can help protect you from nutritional deficiencies and diseases. But when the product name or front label says whole-grain, you may only be talking about a small percent of the product, with the rest being highly refined, fiberless, and almost nutritionless wheat flour. As if that is not enough, a manufacturer can run a grain over a stone grinder and then later run it through a steel roller mill and still call it stone-ground!

Our advice in this deceptive world of food labeling is to look, feel, and taste a bread or flour for coarseness and the presence of a generous amount of whole grains. Also, if whole-grain or whole-wheat is listed first in the ingredient table, you know you are getting the benefit of all the nutritious elements of the original grain, including fiber, in the major portion of the bread or flour. But, even then, if the grains have been pulverized into a fine, light, and fluffy product, the GI may be almost as high as some of the non-whole-wheat products (see Figure 2).

In an effort to help you better understand the rest of labeling and to make you a better *Sugar Busters!* shopper, we have included more information on reading labels. See Figure 13 for two examples of food labels.

Nutritional facts are based on a single recommended serving size (the serving size is on the label). The information provided usually pertains to calories, total fats, saturated fats, cholesterol, sodium, total carbohydrate, fiber, sugars, vitamins, minerals, and "other ingredients." We will discuss each one of these items separately so you can understand their significance.

*Calories* are a basic characteristic of each food source. There are approximately nine calories per gram of fat, seven calories per gram of alcohol, four calories per gram of carbohydrate, and four calories per gram of protein. Obviously, foods with a higher fat content per serving will have more calories than a food with an equal content of carbohydrate or pro-

## Figure 13.

| Sugar Busters!<br>Acceptable | Sugar Busters!<br>Unacceptable |
|---|---|

### Nutrition Facts

Serving Size 1/3 cup (199g)
Servings Per Container 2½

**Amount Per Serving**

| **Calories** 20 | Calories from Fat 0 |
|---|---|

| | **% Daily Value*** |
|---|---|
| **Total Fat** 0g | **0%** |
| Saturated Fat 0g | **0%** |
| **Cholesterol** 0mg | **0%** |
| **Sodium** 420mg | **17%** |
| **Total Carbohydrate** 3g | **1%** |
| Dietary Fiber 1g | **5%** |
| Sugars less than 1g | |
| **Protein** 2g | |

| Vitamin A 6% | • | Vitamin C 15% |
|---|---|---|
| Calcium 0% | • | Iron 2% |

*Percent Daily Values are based on 2,000 calorie diet

**INGREDIENTS:** CUT GREEN ASPARAGUS, WATER, SALT

### Nutrition Facts

Serving Size 2 cookies (33g)
Servings Per Container about 10

**Amount Per Serving**

| **Calories** 150 | Calories from Fat 60 |
|---|---|

| | **% Daily Value*** |
|---|---|
| **Total Fat** 6g | **9%** |
| Saturated Fat 3.5g | **10%** |
| **Cholesterol** 35mg | **11%** |
| **Sodium** 110mg | **8%** |
| **Total Carbohydrate** 22g | **7%** |
| Dietary Fiber less than 1g | **4%** |
| Sugars 9g | |
| **Protein** 2g | |

| Vitamin A 4% | • | Vitamin C 0% |
|---|---|---|
| Calcium 2% | • | Iron 5% |

* Percent Daily Values are based on a 2,000 calorie diet. Your daily values may be higher or lower depending on your calorie needs.

| | Calories | 2000 | 2,500 |
|---|---|---|---|
| Total Fat | Less than | 65g | 80g |
| Sat. Fat | Less than | 20g | 25g |
| Cholesterol | Less than | 300mg | 300mg |
| Sodium | Less than | 2,400mg | 2,400mg |
| Total Carbohydrate | | 300g | 375g |
| Dietary Fiber | | 25g | 30g |

Calories per gram:
Fat 9  •  Carbohydrate 4  •  Protein 4

**INGREDIENTS:** BUTTER, BLEACHED ENRICHED WHEAT FLOUR [CONTAINS BLEACHED WHEAT FLOUR, WHEAT FLOUR, NIACIN, REDUCED IRON, THIAMINE (VITAMIN B₁), MONONITRATES, RIBOFLAVIN (VITAMIN B₂), FOLIC ACID]; ROLLED OATS, SUGAR, FANCY MOLASSES, BROWN SUGAR, MILK, LEAVENING (BAKING POWDER, BAKING SODA); SALT, NATURAL FLAVOR tein. Remember, calories are calculated from the basic components of the food product and, by themselves, do not indicate the important following nutritional information.

*Total fats* are an important component of many food products. With the exception of meats, milk, and oils, fat grams should be low—approximately one to three grams per serving. Lean, trimmed meats should have no more than five grams of fat per serving. Low-fat cheese should have no more than one to two grams of fat per serving. Two-percent milk should have slightly less than five grams per eight-ounce glass. Products with a normally high fat content such as cooking oils, may contain as much as seven to nine grams of fat, but the largest percentage of this fat should be poly- or monounsaturated. These are the so-called good fats.

Many products contain trans fats, which are vegetable oils to which additional hydrogen ions have been added during preparation. Trans fats have effects on our bodies similar to saturated animal fats and, when possible, should always be avoided. New federal guidelines on nutritional information hopefully will require that trans fats be listed on nutritional labels. Some common foods that often contain trans fats are margarine, cookies, donuts, pizzas, and fried foods.

Trying to reduce your intake of unnecessary fats, especially saturated fats, is good, healthy, and recommended on *Sugar Busters!* However, we do need some fat for the proper functioning of our bodies. Removing all fat from your diet is not healthy. When it comes to fat, remember moderation. Equally as harmful to us as foods with too much fat are those that are advertised as low or no-fat, which usually means high-sugar. Excessive amounts of added refined sugar as well as excessive amounts of high-glycemic carbohydrates, like white flour, can ultimately be converted to and stored in our bodies as fat.

*Cholesterol* is a component of most meat and dairy products. You should avoid ingesting unnecessary cholesterol, but, in most people, diets containing several hundred milligrams of cholesterol a day are not harmful. Only 40 percent of the ingested cholesterol is actually absorbed into our systems. But, when given a choice of different foods in a particular category, choose the ones with the lower cholesterol contents.

*Sodium* is salt and is added to enhance flavor or to cut the sweet taste in foods containing an over-abundance of sugars. While some sodium is good for our daily diet, too much is harmful. The conventionally recommended daily allowance (RDA) of sodium is 2,400 milligrams. This is only about one-half of a teaspoon! If you exercise daily, ask your doctor if you need more than the RDA for salt. See the paragraph on vitamins below.

*"Carbohydrates"* basically refer to all the sugar, either naturally occurring or added, in a particular

food product. Fruits have a high content of fruit sugar (fructose), and milk products have high content of milk sugar (galactose). But most carbohydrates are in the form of grains or starches and, as such, have very little simple sugars or "sugars" that are required to be added to the Nutrition Facts label. With the exception of fruits and dairy products, carbohydrate products, including grains and cereals, should contain as little refined sugar as possible and in any case, no more than five grams of "sugars" per serving. A high "sugars" content—except in fruits and milk—is an important warning sign that the product is unacceptable on *Sugar Busters!* and probably has too much added refined sugar.

Why do we differentiate the "fruit" and "milk" sugars? If we use glucose as the 100 percent GI standard, sucrose rates 65 on that scale, milk or galactose sugar is 43, and fructose (fruit sugar) has only a GI of 22. So three grams of sucrose, table sugar, gives a glycemic reaction approximately three times that of three grams of fructose, and three grams of fructose gives a GI 50 percent lower than three grams of milk sugar. As you can see, when trying to control blood insulin levels, blood sugar, and weight, eating the natural sugars in fruit, dairy products, and low-glycemic vegetables is preferable to eating sucrose. Additionally, you get no vitamins, minerals, and other important elements from table sugar.

*Fiber* is an extremely important component of

many carbohydrates. The higher the fiber content of a food product, the healthier it is for you. As a generality, the high-fiber fruits and vegetables are low-glycemic and they are also the fruit and vegetables that are richest in antioxidants. The incidence of colon cancer as well as some other medical problems is reduced in those people eating a high-fiber diet. You should eat at least twenty-five to thirty grams of fiber daily. Green leafy vegetables and whole-grain products are excellent sources of our fiber requirements.

*Proteins* may be derived from either plant or animal sources. Most of your protein will come from meat and dairy products, but grains and vegetables are also a good source. All balanced diets should contain sufficient protein for your basic daily requirements. It is important to note that two of the essential amino acids (lysine and methionine) are best derived from animal protein and thus the optimal diet will contain some animal or fish protein.

*Vitamins and minerals* are both important to the proper functioning of our bodies. A well-balanced diet as suggested by the authors of *Sugar Busters!* contains all the essential vitamins and minerals required by a healthy person. A glass of freshly squeezed orange or grapefruit juice contains as much potassium as a ripe banana. Most foods contain more than an adequate amount of sodium. You should be careful about adding additional salt when cooking or seasoning, especially if you have a heart of blood pressure problem. If you are concerned about your daily intake of sufficient vitamins and minerals, a good commercially available vitamin with minerals, such as Theragran-M and Centrum, more than ensures adequate daily intake of these substances. Please note that some of these multivitamins still contain, at the time of this writing, more than the recommended daily allowance of vitamin A, which has recently been lowered to 700 IUs (international units).

*Other ingredients* are supplements and additives that processors have included in the preparation of their food products. These include high-fructose corn syrup, maltodextrin, dextrose, xylol, maltose, malt, isomalt, hydrolyzed starch, hydrolyzed rice starch, syrups, honey, and brown sugar. On the label, they are listed in order, from the largest to the smallest amount. Although some of these terms may not be familiar to you, they are all disguised sugars. They have been added for the purpose of enhancing the taste or thickening the particular product. Their ultimate effect will be to raise your insulin levels and create more fat on your body. Sugar alcohols, such as sorbitol, and maltotal, which are often present in low-sugar diet ice creams, may cause gastrointestinal irritation and diarrhea if ingested in large amounts. Although it is often difficult to avoid these additives altogether, every effort should be made to select those products that have as few and as little of these supplements as possible.

In summary, interpreting nutritional facts on food-product labels is not easy, but having a little knowledge about what this information means can make your shopping on *Sugar Busters!* much more successful.

# 21 | Lifetime Meal Plans

Rather than a seven-, fourteen-, or thirty-day meal plan, we have simply included suggestions from which you can select meals for a lifetime of healthy eating. We do recommend that you vary your selections from time to time to take advantage of the full range of natural vitamins, minerals, and other nutrients that Mother Nature has made available.

By putting together your own combinations for meals, you can optimize shopping and the timely consumption of foods that have a limited shelf or refrigerator life. You also can satisfy your current cravings from the extensive list of foods allowed on the *Sugar Busters!* lifestyle. Recipes for many of the foods can be found in the "Super Foods" chapter of this book or in the *Sugar Busters! Quick and Easy Cookbook* or the original hardcover *Sugar Busters! Cut Sugar to Trim Fat*. Recipes from many of your cookbooks can be modified to be acceptable on the *Sugar Busters!* lifestyle. Some of the longer-shelf-life foods are useful to have in your well-stocked pantry, as discussed in Chapter 12.

We hope you enjoy putting together the various individual items that will best suit your individual palate.

## Breakfast Suggestions from Which to Choose

Fruit before: cantaloupe, honeydew, orange, grapefruit, grapes, kiwi, peach, pear, blueberries, raspberries, strawberries, or blackberries

Eggs; poached, scrambled, or fried over medium-low heat in olive or canola oil, butter, or non-hydrogenated margarine

Cheese omelet; onion, mushroom, and tomato omelet; ham and cheese omelet; bell pepper and onion omelet; smoked salmon omelet

Canadian bacon or smoked fish

Whole-grain toast (two-slice limit)

Breakfast cereals (as whole-grain as possible and with no sugar added)

Oatmeal with milk, an artificial or natural sweetener (aspartame, saccharin, stevia, fructose, or Trutina Dulcem), and some of the berries listed above

If you like, you can simply eat a breakfast of one or more of the fruits.

## Lunch Suggestions from Which to Choose

Sandwiches of whole-grain wheat, rye, pumpernickel, or whole-wheat pita bread, either tuna salad, egg salad, chicken salad, roast beef or grilled chicken. Also a reuben sandwich with dark rye bread and sauerkraut is good, as is a vegetarian sandwich or whole-wheat pita pocket with avocados, alfalfa sprouts, shaved carrots, cucumbers, and other vegetables. Any entrée-type salad that does not contain potatoes, sweetened salad dressings, or battered and fried meats or vegetables is okay, as well as a large fruit salad. You may also eat any of the dinner meals if you prefer your large meal at lunch.

## Dinner Suggestions from Which to Choose

Skillet- or broiler-grilled salmon, tuna, chicken, steak, lamb, pork, ground meat, wild game, or other fish. Also roasted beef, pork, lamb, chicken, or wild game. Serve with at least two of the following fruits or vegetables plus a green salad: avocado, asparagus, broccoli, Brussels sprouts, cauliflower, bell peppers, squash, zucchini, eggplant, mushrooms, cabbage, onions, tomatoes, celery, sweet potatoes, beans (pinto, black, red, navy, or garbanzo), green beans, green peas, black-eyed peas, snow peas, spinach, kale, mustard or collard greens. Another accompaniment could be whole-grain pasta with a no-sugar-added sauce.

## Snack Suggestions from Which to Choose

A piece of fruit, a handful of nuts, a cup of berries, peanut butter on a celery stick or three or four whole-wheat crackers, such as Triscuits, some raw vegetables (broccoli, cauliflower, carrots, radishes, celery, bell peppers, squash, zucchini, or cherry or grape tomatoes) dipped in a no-sugar-added salad dressing or spicy salt, hard-boiled egg, half an avocado with lemon juice and salt, a piece of cheese, ripe or green olives, cocktail onions or shallots (if you work alone!), a few bites of leftover meats or vegetables.

## Drink Suggestions from Which to Choose

Coffee, tea, green tea, milk, or water. If you must occasionally drink soda, drink a clear diet soda (it will not contain phosphoric acid, as do colas).

## Dessert Suggestions

The *Sugar Busters!* lifestyle should help diminish your cravings for refined sugars (your "sweet tooth"). We understand, however, what you will likely eat a dessert from time to time.

A few nuts can often satisfy the craving for a sweet dessert. It is probably the fat that adds the extra satisfaction from eating nuts. Fortunately, the fat in nuts is primarily monounsaturated, heart-healthy fat. One or two squares of high-cocoa content chocolate (60 percent or greater cocoa) is acceptable, since the sugar content is usually lower than that of low-cocoa chocolate. Modest portions of no-sugar-added ice cream are also acceptable if you have eaten a low-glycemic meal that does not contain red meat.

## 22 | The Plateaus

Most people who change their way of eating to the *Sugar Busters!* lifestyle experience an initial period of rapid weight loss, which can be two to three or even five or more pounds in the first two weeks. The rate of weight loss will vary from individual to individual for many different reasons. These initial variations and subsequent variations in rate of loss can be caused by differing rates of metabolism; by how much or how little weight one needs to lose; by how closely one adheres to the new way of eating; by how much food is consumed (the temptation to eat a lot is great when you see the needle on the scale dropping despite the rather high caloric intake); by the metabolic effect of medications, birth control pills, or hormone replacement therapy; or by whether one has a medical condition, such as a thyroid disorder.

One thing is certain, however—the rate of weight loss will not be on a constant, even, descending slope. After an initial weight loss of five, ten, or even fifteen pounds, you may experience a plateau, a temporary cessation of weight loss, even though you have not changed your diet or exercise program.

If you are lucky, it may only be a "tilted plateau," or a slowing of weight loss for a period of time. How long will a plateau last, and how many will you experience? Again, it will vary from individual to individual. Based on reports from many of the followers of the *Sugar Busters!* lifestyle, plateaus can last from one week to as many as six weeks before weight loss or a higher rate of weight loss resumes. People who need to lose ten pounds or so and lose it all in the first few weeks may never experience a plateau. For those needing to lose many tens or over a hundred pounds, it is likely several plateaus of short duration, or even a "six-weeker," will be experienced.

Do not let the plateaus discourage you. They are common and they will be temporary until you reach your natural weight. How can you determine your natural weight? Can it be read from a chart of height, weight, and age? No, not precisely. Many of us are simply built differently. Some have small bones, small waists, and small muscles. Others have larger bones, larger waists, and larger muscles. Ditto for people of any height. All that said, using a target of a Body Mass Index less than 25 is usually reasonable.

A good rule of thumb once was to go back and look at a picture of your body around age twenty-one to twenty-five and assume you could approach (but probably not reach) that weight again through following a program of good diet and exercise. We say it *once was* a good rule of thumb because, a few decades back, the average person was much thinner at age twenty-one to twenty-five than an average person is today. The earlier generations ate better and got more exercise. They ate fewer highly refined foods and far less added sugar, and they exercised more because of fewer convenience devices (including the lack of a car for every member of the family) and had fewer attractions that can entertain one without any physical exercise participation, such as watching television or operating a computer. But today, a high percentage of our young adults are overweight, and a significant percentage are already obese.

Since our gene pools have not had time to change dramatically in just a few decades, we believe the "once was" target can still be used even for the younger generation.

We suggest you look at a picture of your parents or grandparents when they were in their early to mid-twenties. Use that to pick a reasonable target for your desired weight and eat your way to it. The beauty of the *Sugar Busters!* lifestyle is that you will not feel deprived of good, filling foods or of a tremendous variety of foods while you eat your way to success.

# 23 | Why <u>Sugar Busters!</u>

The bookstores are now carrying many best-selling diet books that recommend many of the things that were included in our original *Sugar Busters! Cut Sugar to Trim Fat*. We are happy to see that people are waking up to the fact that diets loaded with high-glycemic carbohydrates have been causing rampant weight gain and its associated health problems.

However, the most common criticism we hear about most of these books is that they contain too much detailed biochemistry or require too much counting and measuring for the average reader.

A diet of low-glycemic carbohydrates is not necessarily the same as a low-carbohydrate diet. Our ancestors, who successfully got us here, did not have high-glycemic carbohydrates to eat, and they certainly did not know what vitamins, minerals, and other nutrients their foods contained. Neither did they count their carbohydrates or protein or fat grams. As reported in our earlier books and meal plans, we think a diet should have carbohydrates as its major source of calories. That content can exceed 50 percent if all the carbohydrates are of the high-fiber, low-glycemic type. Eat a good variety of them and you will be well on your way to satisfying your various nutritional requirements. Just keep it simple, and "start out like you can hold out."

Regarding the current debate on high-protein, high-fat diets, like Atkins, versus low-fat or nonfat diets, like Ornish, we see significant advantages of eating the *Sugar Busters!* way.

First, the *Sugar Busters!* lifestyle encourages a diet in which at least 40 percent of calories come from high-fiber, low-glycemic carbohydrates. These carbohydrates deliver huge amounts of vitamins, minerals, antioxidants, and trace elements that are not present in the meats consumed in an Atkins-like diet.

Second, the *Sugar Busters!* lifestyle provides about 30 percent of calories from protein, including some animal protein, which provides the building blocks for optimum cell formation. The lifestyle also suggests that about 30 percent of calories come from fat, which contains the fatty acids that are needed for optimum health and nutrition. The animal proteins are not available in a vegetarian-type or vegan diet.

Third, the *Sugar Busters!* lifestyle is a healthy and balanced plan that provides not only the necessary variety of vitamins and minerals from natural foods but also the satisfaction and enjoyment not consistently available from the more extreme diets.

Fourth, the *Sugar Busters!* lifestyle is simple and

easy to follow. There is no initial period of crash dieting required. There are no food exchange values to
count. There is not much high-tech biochemistry
included, which can confuse the average person.

The following paragraphs contain brief comments
on some of the other diets currently available in
bookstores around the country.

Dr. Atkins certainly deserves credit for being the
early champion, in the modern era, of eating more
protein and fat as a weight-loss tool. He pointed out
many of the pitfalls of high-carbohydrate diets. We
don't understand why he so severely limits all types
of carbohydrates, which then requires the consumption of expensive vitamin and mineral supplements
(which he is happy to sell you). As has been demonstrated by the legions of *Sugar Busters!* followers,
weight loss and nutritious eating can be achieved
simultaneously by including the low-glycemic, high-
fiber, natural carbohydrates in one's daily eating plan.
And the latter plan can be followed enjoyably for a
lifetime. *Sugar Busters!* is <u>NOT</u> an Atkins-like way
of eating.

Dean Ornish's diet *(Eat More, Weigh Less)* may be
of some benefit to people with severe blood chemistry or cardiovascular problems, but it is certainly
not a natural way of eating. No meat, no oils, no
nuts! How did our ancestors get us here? What did
they eat in the long winter months when the fruits
and vegetables did not grow? Only meat, seeds, and

nuts were available for survival except for those peoples who lived very near the equator. We also note that Ornish's last no-no is sugar, which, with the significant calorie restrictions of his diet, may just be what causes the weight loss that can occur on his diet.

*The Zone*, by Dr. Barry Sears, contains a lot of good information and advice, but it also contains so much biochemistry that the average person easily can get confused as to what causes what. Also, many of his followers tire of the constant counting required to stay "in the zone." Again, you can bet our forefathers never worried about a "zone." Since they only had low-glycemic fruits, vegetables, and whole grains available, they just naturally stayed "in the zone," the way one can today by simply following the *Sugar Busters!* lifestyle.

The *Protein Power* diet is well presented and well researched, and it is undoubtedly of use to professional nutritionists and dietitians. However, the book contains so much biochemistry that it loses its chance to be an easily understandable and easy-to-follow guide for the average citizen.

*The Carbohydrate Addict's Diet*, which allows you to pig out prior to bedtime, just doesn't make sense. Most of a person's cholesterol is made at night, and the natural metabolism also slows with the lack of physical movement, so why say it is all right to stoke the fire by having a huge evening meal? Why not just have people eat the right carbohydrates (high-fiber, low-glycemic) in significant quantities and let it go at that?

Dr. Andrew Weil says in *Eating Well for Optimal Health* that it is okay to be fat, and we understand the point he is trying to make. But when the national statistics so clearly indicate the myriad diseases associated with being fat, we don't think people should be told it is okay to be fat, even if they would love to hear it. They will read that and conveniently forget or ignore many of the other important points in his book.

While Jennie Brand-Miller and colleagues have certainly participated in a lot of valuable glycemic index measurements in Australia, the conclusions in her book *The Glycemic Revolution* are that eating sugar, high-glycemic white potatoes, and other such foods is okay. That can seem like great news for Americans, who are consuming an average of almost fifty teaspoons of added almost nutritionless refined sugar per person per day and experiencing epidemic problems with obesity, diabetes, and related diseases! Even though she indicates from time to time that people should eat low-glycemic meals and makes the point that a low-glycemic-index piece of meat consumed with a very high-glycemic carbohydrate (like a white potato) will moderate the overall glycemic response, she misses the point that the same piece of meat consumed with a low-glycemic-index carbohydrate will give a still lower glycemic response and also deliver necessary vitamins and minerals, producing even greater weight loss or control.

Following are some summary quotes by Brand-Miller and colleagues: "Low GI diets can help people lose weight." "To make the change to a low GI diet use more pastas and rice in place of potatoes," and then on the very next page "Bread and potatoes are rich in carbohydrate and therefore among the best foods you can eat to help you lose weight." On the same page is "Some starch, like that in potatoes, is digested in a flash, causing a greater rise in blood sugar than many sugar-containing foods."

"Sugar has no unique role in causing diabetes." "Foods that produce high blood sugar levels may increase the risk of diabetes." Well, according to her own GI tables, sugar is not a low GI food, and also, refined sugar is usually associated with highly processed flours that have a high GI value.

"Diets high in sugar are less nutritious. Not true. Sugar (from a range of sources including dairy products and fruit) often has higher levels of micronutrients." Here Brand-Miller is swiching back and forth on whether she is talking about refined sugar or about the natural sugars found in fruits, grains, and vegetables. Are you confused yet? So are we.

The *Sugar Busters!* bottom line is this: why encourage consumption of refined sugar and high-glycemic carbohydrates at all in light of the fact that the resulting obesity has done so much harm to so many people?

If you want confirmation that it is not the consumption of fat that has been making us fat, consider the Duke University six-month trial of the Atkins Diet versus the American Heart Association's Low-Fat Step 1 Diet. The Atkins Diet contained 60 percent fat and beat the AHA diet on every count: weight loss, HDL (good) cholesterol improvement, and reduction in triglycerides. So why not just choose the Atkins Diet? As we have said, you will lose the benefit of the known and yet undetected beneficial elements that are present in the low-glycemic fruits and vegetables. That is why we firmly believe that the *Sugar Busters!* lifestyle is BEYOND ATKINS!

In summary, if you follow the general principles in *Sugar Busters! Cut Sugar to Trim Fat*, you can enjoy your meals without counting your "zone" portions or your calories (within reason). If you get the sugar and other nutrients that your body requires from the nutrition-filled, low-glycemic carbohydrates, you won't get fat and unhealthy in the first place.

# 24 | Alternative Sweeteners

There are now several alternative sweeteners on the market. Some are nutritive and some are non-nutritive. Nearly all are commonly referred to as artificial sweeteners. Some are not found in nature, while others are concentrated forms of natural sugars. One, not yet approved by the Food and Drug Administration (FDA) to be marketed as an artificial sweetener, is actually a naturally occurring herb. All of these sweeteners have one thing in common: they do not have a fattening or blood-sugar-elevating effect like sucrose, brown sugar, molasses, honey, or corn syrup. The purpose of replacing these "natural" sugars is to provide a sweet product that does not have a fattening or blood-sugar-elevating effect like the natural sugars.

The most common question asked about any of these sweeteners is whether they are safe. Our survey of the technical literature indicates that the FDA is quite thorough and conservative in its approach to approving any new sweetener. The FDA also has a history of performing continuing studies on these sweeteners in response to almost any new question or accusation that may arise. Cyclamates, for example, have been taken off the market in response to some fairly weak indications that very high dosages of the sweeteners, when given to animals, caused potential problems. We acknowledge the need to be conservative when it comes to approving new sweeteners and concur that the testing should continue. We are satisfied, however, that the products currently approved by the FDA can be considered safe unless and until new scientific studies prove otherwise.

Remember that, as with almost any substance, it is the size of the dose that counts. Even table sugar, consumed in huge quantities, can have a harmful effect on many people's bodies by helping to cause obesity, diabetes, and many other related diseases.

Should you just eliminate added sweeteners of any type to achieve the optimum diet? Ideally, yes. Practically, no. First, you cannot dodge them all; they are in most of the manufactured products on the market. Second, now that humankind has been exposed to the pleasures of eating something (besides fruit) that tastes sweet, it is very unlikely that most people will voluntarily forgo that pleasure. We do recommend that you eliminate as much added sugar or alternative sweetener as you can and try to satisfy your desire for sweets by getting them from the natural sugars that are present in fruits and vegetables.

Let's discuss some of the alternative sweeteners that are on the market today.

*Aspartame.* Primarily marketed as Equal or Nutra-Sweet, aspartame was approved by the FDA in 1981. It is made up of two amino acids, aspartic acid and phenylalanine, and is digested and metabolized in the same manner as other ingested proteins. Aspartame is approximately 200 times sweeter than an equal amount of table sugar, and although it is technically a nutritive sweetener, so little is required that it, or the slight amounts of other additives such as maltodextrin or dextrose, have an insignificant effect on blood sugar.

The FDA says aspartame is one of the most thoroughly studied sweeteners on the market. The FDA has yet to substantiate any of the thousands of accusations that have been leveled by various individuals or groups, some of who may have motives to remove all alternative sweeteners from the market. The one potential problem that was acknowledged early on is that the phenylalanine in aspartame can be bad for anyone having a rare hereditary disease called phenylketonuria (PKU); these people should avoid anything containing phenylalanine. Also, aspartame does not hold up well when exposed to high heat.

*Saccharin.* Primarily marketed as Sweet 'N Low,

saccharin came on the market decades ago, before FDA approval was necessary. It cannot be absorbed by the body and is thus a non-nutritive sweetener. Saccharin is 300 times sweeter than an equal amount of table sugar. It was found to cause bladder cancer in rats that were fed huge amounts of saccharin, but since it has been used for so long with no apparent problems arising in humans, the FDA has allowed saccharin to remain on the market.

*Acesulfame potassium (Acesulfame-K)*. Primarily marketed as Sunette or Sweet One, this sweetener is in hundreds of sugar-free products, including some diet drinks and chewing gums. It is approximately 200 times sweeter than an equal amount of table sugar. The FDA has declared the product safe. Of course, it should not be used by anyone on a potassium-limited diet or anyone with any allergies related to potassium-bearing products.

*Sucralose*. Primarily marketed as Splenda, Sucralose was approved by the FDA in 1998. It is estimated to be approximately 600 times sweeter than table sugar. Sucralose is made from sugar, but the chemical alteration means that it contains molecules that are too large for it to be absorbed into the body; it is thus a non-nutritive sweetener. It can be utilized for products requiring cooking or freezing.

*Fructose*. Fructose is a natural fruit sugar, but it has a glycemic index of only 22, about one-third that of table sugar. It causes a lower elevation in blood sugar and a lower requirement for insulin than an equivalent amount of table sugar. For those who insist on a natural sweetener, it is a reasonable substitute for table sugar. There are also sweeteners derived from fruit sugars or fruit concentrates, such as kiwi, dates, etc., which are gaining in popularity.

*Stevia* (Stevia rebaudiana). Stevia is an herb that is native to South America and has been used there as a sweetener for centuries. The Japanese have used stevia for over thirty years. It has not yet been approved by the FDA as an artificial sweetener and can only be marketed in health food stores as a dietary supplement. Stevia is marketed in both a powdered and liquid form and can require some testing by the individual user to determine how much is required to replace a given amount of sugar. It is, however, another natural sweetener from which to choose.

What's the bottom line on this group of alternative sweeteners? They all impart a lower glycemic effect on our bodies than table sugar, and this helps control insulin and thus weight as well as the effects of diabetes. None of the alternative sweeteners make any significant nutritive contribution, but the same is true for nutritionless, empty-calorie table sugar, which does cause a significant rise in blood sugar. We agree with the American Heart Association's recommendation that artificial sweeteners can be used by diabetics and persons on a weight-loss diet. We do believe that the alternative sweeteners should be used in moderation and in conjunction with an otherwise healthy diet containing ample amounts of low-glycemic, high-fiber carbohydrates, like those recommended in *Sugar Busters!*

## 25 | To Drink or Not to Drink

Research on the effects of alcohol consumption has increased significantly in the last several years. There is broad acceptance in the American and international medical community that the consumption of moderate amounts of alcohol will, in fact, lower the mortality rate of drinkers versus nondrinkers (see Figure 8, page 81).

For those of you who do not drink, we are not recommending that you start, because an excess consumption of alcohol causes many more problems than a moderate consumption appears to help.

Many are extolling, in particular, the greater benefit of wine rather than beer or hard liquor. European medical researchers have led this effort. Noted French epidemiologist Serge Renaud claims, "It's well documented that a moderate intake of alcohol prevents heart disease by as much as 50 percent" and further, that "there is no other drug that's as efficient as the moderate intake of alcohol."[1]

Research by epidemiologist Morten Gronbaek of Denmark concludes that consuming alcohol in the form of wine versus beer or hard liquor is important in lowering the risk of dying from cancer.[2]

Other Europeans currently active in research on the effects of alcohol consumption are researchers Serenello Rotondo and Giovanni de Gaetano of Italy, Jean-Marc Orgogozo and Joseph Vercanteren of France, and Elias Castaras of Greece. The collective wisdom of these researchers confirms the benefits of some alcohol in one's diet, and several believe that the polyphenols and bioflavonoids (both strong antioxidants) in red wine make it particularly effective in fighting problems such as cardiovascular disease, prostate and breast cancer, and dementia, including Alzheimer's disease.

Dr. Jean-Marc Orgogozo, chairman of the Department of Neurology at University Hospital Pellegrin in Bordeaux, France, has done studies on the effect of the drinking habits of 3,777 people age sixty-five and older. Dr. Orgogozo found that of the 60 percent who drank regularly (95 percent of their consumption was red wine), the moderate drinkers had an 80 percent reduction in dementia and a 75 percent reduction in Alzheimer's disease after the first five years of the study compared with the nondrinkers. As they aged, the benefit lessened somewhat, but they still showed a 50 percent reduction in the incidence of Alzheimer's disease eight years into the study. Dr. Orgogozo defined moderate consumption as two to three 4½-ounce glasses of wine per day for women and three to four glasses for men.[3] Other researchers generally define moderate consumption as two to three 3.5-ounce glasses of wine per day.

Since many of the studies have shown significant statistical improvements in mortality rates for moderate drinkers and further encouraging results in laboratory and animal studies, we suggest that you stay tuned for additional reports in these and related areas. Remember, however, we are not recommending that you start drinking alcohol if you do not drink. Many of the cardiovascular benefits can be derived by taking aspirin and drinking a glass of purple grape juice.

You can lose weight more quickly if you do not drink alcohol at all. But if you do continue to drink in moderation, avoid beer and sugar-laden mixers.

Note that while researchers see positive health effects from drinking moderate amounts of alcohol, the situation reverses itself quite quickly once alcohol consumption increases. Not only does excessive drinking endanger your own health but it can also cause both heartache and physical harm to those you are around or who are on the road with you.

# 26 | Fat Versus Low-Fat Diets and Products

The "eat some fat" versus "eat low-fat" debate is finally getting some national attention, and we are pleased to see this happen. The clinical evidence for the health benefits of eating very restricted amounts of fat has been lacking. The same lack of evidence exists for the health benefits of diets very high in carbohydrates. The evidence indicates that while many of our forebears ate high-fat diets, they, as well as those who ate near-vegetarian diets or a seasonal mixture of both, survived and ultimately outperformed the other species on earth. It has only been in recent history that we have been told to severely restrict our intake of fat.

An article in *Science* magazine did a good job of revealing that the government's decision to recommend a significant restriction on fat consumption was a political decision rather than one based on clinical or scientific evidence.[1] What is surprising is how quickly and how thoroughly the government and the general populace bought the "fat is bad" message, resulting in a 16 percent drop in fat grams consumed.[2]

The results of this political decision, made twenty-five years ago, has had many ramifications:

- A huge, multibillion-dollar industry built on low-fat products has been established.
- The fats eliminated from the products have often been replaced by nutritionless refined sugars and highly refined flours.
- Overweight- and obesity-related diseases have become national epidemics and have surely shortened and worsened the lives of millions of people.
- Overweight and obesity epidemics have also affected our children.

A very recent advisory by the American Heart Association said that despite the growing availability and popularity of foods made with fat substitutes, there is no evidence that low- or reduced-fat foods are effective weight loss tools.[3]

For many years, people thought that eating fat increased the risk for breast cancer. New studies are not bearing this out. According to Melanie Polk, director of nutrition at the American Institute for Cancer Research in Washington, D.C., "The research is not as strong as originally thought. . . . The evidence is much stronger for other lifestyle factors."[4] But, as you will see elsewhere, the fatter you become, the higher will be your risk for breast cancer.

"The fat [that we eat] turns to fat" argument has been easily believed by our politicians as well as the general population. As previously mentioned in Chapter 9, the surprising thing is that this "fat is bad" line of thinking was bought almost unanimously by professional nutritionists and dietitians despite evidence in the medical literature and textbooks that it is much easier to convert available carbohydrates to body fat. With our population encouraged for decades to eat very high amounts of all forms of carbohydrates, our bodies have consistently had excess carbohydrates available to be stored as fat.

Since few doctors in America studied nutrition, they, as a group, seldom disputed the nutrition profession's dogma that it is predominantly the fat that turns to fat. As mentioned previously, the two ships (professions) just passed in the night. It would appear that dawn is imminent and that each ship will now see the other and mankind's knowledge regarding what foods work best for people performing at various levels of activity will be significantly advanced.

To obtain the most beneficial effect from the foods we eat, we need some fat in our diets. Fatty acids are necessary for many chemical activities in the body that affect growth, metabolism, manufacture of cell membranes and sex hormones, and transport of the vitamins A, D, E, and K. Fats also add the flavor and texture that provide both pleasure and a feeling of fullness after a meal. The ability to provide the feeling of fullness may be why a few nuts consumed at the end of a meal seem to satisfy the desire for a sugar-laden dessert.

There are three types of fat: monounsaturated, polyunsaturated, and saturated fat. The first two have been demonstrated to have some beneficial effects, such as raising the HDL (good) cholesterol and/or lowering the LDL (bad) cholesterol. The jury is still out on how much saturated fat can be consumed safely over long periods of time. Consumption of saturated fat with a meal of high-glycemic, low-fiber carbohydrates still appears to us to be a risk we need not take unless or until future clinical studies prove otherwise. Saturated fat can average about 10 percent of your calories, but do not consistently overindulge in saturated fat.

We recommend consumption of monounsaturated fats, like the fat in olive oil, avocados, seeds, and nuts. We also recommend the polyunsaturated fats, like those found in cold-water fish, walnuts, and vegetable oils (corn, safflower, and soybean).

In conclusion, reagarding fat, we think that some fat in the diet is beneficial, as it was for our ancestors. A target of 30 percent of total calories from fat (or even 40 percent) is reasonable if most of the fat is monounsaturated and polyunsaturated. However, the carbohydrate content of a diet should always be of low-glycemic and high-fiber fruits, vegetables, and whole-grain products. See Chapter 11 for more discussion on the correct carbohydrates to eat.

# 27 | Conclusion

The *Sugar Busters!* lifestyle is not another high-fat, low-carbohydrate fad diet. The *Sugar Busters!* lifestyle is a balanced, time-tested nutritional lifestyle. It is logical, practical, and reasonable, and involves making healthy and nutritious choices about the foods we eat. The *Sugar Busters!* lifestyle supports removing unnecessary fat, especially too much saturated fat, from our diet. However, we also support eating moderate amounts of lean, trimmed meats, even red meats, which are healthy sources of protein and fat.

Because we recommend avoiding refined sugar and processed grain products, most of you will eat somewhat fewer carbohydrates than you are currently consuming. That is okay, but we do not recommend that you severely restrict carbohydrate consumption. More important, success on the *Sugar Busters!* lifestyle involves a commitment to choosing *correct* carbohydrates. This is a change from mainstream nutritional thinking, which does not differentiate between the metabolic effects of the various carbohydrates.

In health care, transportation, telecommunications, and other fields, tremendous strides have been and are continuing to be made. This has not been so for nutrition and dieting. Our ancestors ate better, often out of necessity, than we do today. How they ate is why our digestive system has evolved to what it is today. Sure, vitamins and other food supplements have improved, and we constantly get to eat a variety of foods with their varying vitamins and minerals. But in general, the way we eat today has caused our health to deteriorate markedly and has prevented a significant increase in life expectancy for middle-aged people. Refining and processing most of what we eat has been an unfortunate nutritional disservice, including the introduction of refined sugar. Our health has suffered as a result.

The evidence for this deterioration has been rather obvious for decades. Most insulin-dependent diabetics gain weight and their cholesterol continues to rise no matter how carefully they follow their doctor's instructions. Many individuals have given up meat entirely only to have their cholesterol levels increase and their vascular disease progress rapidly.

Most nutritionists and dietitians "looked but did not see." Duffy and Montignac began to see. However, because they were not professionally trained in nutrition, many so-called professionals scoffed at or ridiculed them and even suggested they were charlatans.

Most of our body fat is from ingested sugar (carbohydrates), not ingested fat. This is driven by the effects of insulin—aptly proven in the insulin-resistant diabetic who gains still more weight as insulin injections are begun. By modulating insulin secretion through diet, individuals are able to significantly influence body fat, cholesterol, diabetes, and the progression of arteriosclerosis and its subsequent complications. In addition, diet can regulate glucagon secretion, which has additional beneficial effects on fat metabolism that make it easier for the body to utilize previously stored fat.

The world of nutrition is not flat, but round! Previous concepts appeared plausible, but now we have the scientific basis to prove them wrong.

Eating should be an enjoyable and pleasurable experience and contribute to our performance and health. Many have written about refined sugar and its harmful effects. We have taken this premise, verified it by current and historical data, and expanded it to include our belief that insulin is the key. The nutritional and dietary concepts presented in *Sugar Busters!* are consistent with achieving ideal levels of insulin and glucagon secretion.

In addition to pleasuring our palates, the concepts proposed in *Sugar Busters!* should be good news for the cattle ranchers, sheep ranchers, hog farmers, dairy farmers, and egg producers who recently have been much maligned by various health and nutrition groups. These foods are good for us today, just as they were good for our distant ancestors.

The *Sugar Busters!* lifestyle is simple to understand and easy to apply, unlike regimens that call for constant counting and calculating. And, best of all, it is both healthy and satisfying.

With our approach, countless individuals already have experienced weight loss and a reduction in cholesterol, as well as the improvement in performance that is so vital to everyone's success. We feel the same opportunity is available to you by following the recommendations on nutrition and diet we offer in *Sugar Busters!*

*Bon appétit!*

## 28 | Major Restaurants Do <u>Sugar Busters!</u>

This chapter contains recipes from well-known restaurants in many of the major cities in the United States as well as across the globe. Some of the recipes are quick and simple to prepare; for those of you who enjoy spending a creative afternoon in the kitchen, other recipes are more demanding in the acquisition of the ingredients as well as the preparation of the final product.

For readers who do not spend much time in the kitchen and eat out frequently, these recipes can act as a road map for where you might go to order a flavorful and healthy meal, should you happen to be in one of these cities. Many of you have benefited from just reading the many recipes we included in our original book, *Sugar Busters! Cut Sugar to Trim Fat*, that came from major restaurants in New Orleans—and when you came to the city, you could pick your favorite recipe and have it prepared by the local master him- or herself!

For those of you who remain strapped for time but do cook at home, we refer you to our *Sugar*

*Busters! Quick and Easy Cookbook*, which contains flavorful recipes that generally can be prepared in thirty minutes or less.

### Eberhard Mueller, Bayard's (New York City) and Satur Farms (North Fork, Long Island)

#### *Zucchini Noodles*

3 tablespoons extra-virgin olive oil
5 tablespoons thyme leaves, divided
1 teaspoon minced garlic
1½ pounds zucchini, finely julienned
Salt and freshly ground pepper
2 tablespoons minced parsley
1 tablespoon fresh lemon juice

In a large skillet, warm the olive oil. Add 2½ teaspoons of thyme and the garlic and cook over moderate heat for 1 minute. Add the zucchini and cook, stirring occasionally, until it just begins to lose its crunch, about 5 minutes; season it with salt and pepper as it cooks. Transfer the zucchini to a bowl and toss it with the parsley, lemon juice, and the remaining 2½ teaspoons of thyme. Season with salt and pepper and serve warm.

*Serves 4*

### Slow-Roasted Heirloom Tomatoes

6 ripe medium heirloom tomatoes, preferably a mix
   of red, yellow, and green
2 cloves garlic, finely chopped
6 sprigs of thyme, leaves removed and finely
   chopped
Salt and freshly ground pepper
1/2 cup extra-virgin olive oil, plus extra to oil pan
1 tablespoon sherry vinegar

Preheat the oven to 250°F.

In a large saucepan of boiling water, blanch the
tomatoes for 30 seconds. Remove from the water
with a slotted spoon or strainer and immediately
chill in a bowl of ice water to stop the cooking.
The skins will slip right off. Cut the tomatoes in
half, crosswise. Gently squeeze each half to remove seeds.

Oil a 12-by-8-inch or 14-inch oval baking and
sprinkle with half of the garlic and thyme. Season
liberally with salt and pepper. Arrange the tomato
halves, cut sides up, in the dish and baste with
the remaining oil. Season generously with salt
and pepper and sprinkle with the remaining garlic
and thyme and the sherry vinegar.

Bake the tomatoes for 2 1/2 to 3 hours. When done,
they will be soft and just starting to caramelize but
should still hold their shape. Spoon the pan juices

up over the tomatoes and serve from the baking dish.

*Serves 6*

*Originally from the Black Forest of Germany, Eberhard Mueller worked for three years at the three-star Michelin restaurant L' Archestrate. He then opened the famed Le Bernardin with Gilbert LeCoze and was awarded four stars from the* New York Times. *He later became chef of Lutece after Andre Soltner's retirement and is currently the executive chef at Bayard's in downtown Manhattan. He and his wife, Paulette Satur, own Satur Farms on the North Fork of Long Island, where they grow specialty salads, leafy vegetables, heirloom tomatoes, root vegetables, and herbs and are committed to organic farming.*

## Charlie Socher, Café Matou (Chicago, Illinois)

### *Bequet au Four*
### *Roast Lamb Shanks*

4 lamb shanks
Salt and pepper to taste
2 tablespoons dried herbes de provence
4 garlic heads, cut in half

4 onions, peeled and quartered
1 cup white wine
1 cup beef, chicken, or other meat stock
2 anchovy filets, chopped
Zest of 1 lemon
Chopped parsley and lemon wedges for garnish

Preheat the over to 400° F.

Salt and pepper shanks and dust with dried herbes de provence. Place the shanks in a roasting pan and cover; roast for 30 to 40 minutes.

Remove shanks from oven; drain liquid in the pan into a saucepan and reserve.

Add the garlic, onions, white wine, stock, anchovies, and lemon zest to the shanks in the roasting pan and cover. Return the pan to the oven; reduce heat to 325°F., and roast for 1 1/2 hours.

Meanwhile, skim the fat from the reserved liquid; simmer over low heat until liquid is reduced by 1/4. Add this concentrated liquid to that in the roasting pan.

Adjust the seasoning, and serve shanks garnished with chopped parsley and lemon wedges.

*Serves 4.*

*A native Chicagoan and fomer professor of economics, Charlie Socher moved to Paris in 1981 to pursue his cooking career. There he apprenticed at many fine restaurants, including two Michelin-*

*rated restaurants. He then returned to Chicago where he joined the kitchens of such restaurants as Ambria, The Chardonnay, Chez Chazz, Brett's, and Zaven's. He opened Café Matou in 1997 and the restaurant has earned raves from* The Chicago Tribune, Bon Appetit, Chicago *magazine, and* Gault-Millau.

### Franklin Becker, Capitale (New York City)

*Cauliflower-Leek Potage*

2 heads cauliflower
3 leeks, white parts only
2 cloves garlic
1/2 cup ghee (clarified butter)
2 teaspoons madras curry powder
salt and white pepper to taste

Cut the cauliflower and white leeks into equal pieces and place in a pot with the garlic. Add enough cold water to just cover the vegetables. Bring to a boil; reduce heat and let simmer for one hour.

Meanwhile, in a small saucepan over medium heat, melt the ghee. Add the curry powder and remove from the heat being sure not to burn the curry. Strain through a fine mesh strainer and keep warm.

Add the vegetables to a blender, reserving the water in which the vegetables were cooked. Add some of the vegetable water to the blender and process till velvety smooth. While still blending, slowly add the curry butter to the vegetable mixture. Season to taste with salt and pepper and adjust the consistency of the soup if necessary with the remaining vegetable liquid.

Serve hot with sweet-potato chips if desired for texture and contrasting flavors.

*Serves 8*

*After graduating from the Culinary Institute of America, Franklin Becker held chef positions at Mesa Grill, The Penn Club, and the James Beard House. He was the executive chef at Local, where he and his cooking received rave reviews from the media and critics alike. He served as private chef to Revlon magnate Ronald O. Perelman. He is currently executive chef at Capitale, a new restaurant in New York City.*

# Bob Waggoner, Charleston Grill
## (Charleston, South Carolina)

### *Chilled Charleston Heirloom Tomato and Goat Cheese Soup*

$8^{1}/_{2}$ large yellow tomatoes, quartered
3 to 4 large onions, quartered
$2^{1}/_{2}$ cups sliced shallots,
7 garlic cloves
3 to 4 cups Napa Valley Verjus (or $^{1}/_{4}$ cup fresh lemon juice)
$1^{3}/_{4}$ tablespoon Kosher salt
$1^{1}/_{4}$ tablespoon fresh ground white pepper
3 to 4 seeded yellow bell peppers, chopped
$^{1}/_{3}$ cup olive oil
1 pound fresh crumbled goat cheese
1 bunch fresh cilantro, for garnish
1 cucumber, seeded and diced fine, for garnish

In a large mixing bowl, combine the tomatoes, onions, shallots, garlic, verjus or lemon juice, salt, pepper, and bell peppers. Feed this mixture into a blender in small batches, processing as you go.

When all of the vegetable mixture has been blended, slowly add the olive oil while still processing.

Allow soup to chill in the refrigetator for one hour.

When ready to serve, ladle into bowls and evenly

distribute the goat cheese over each serving. Garnish with the cilantro and cucumber.

*Serves 20*

### Stuffed Parma Prosciutto with Goat Cheese, Roasted Pecans, and Sunflower Sprouts in a Sherry Vinegar and Virgin Pecan Oil Vinaigrette

DRESSING

1/3 cup sherry vinegar
2 ounces virgin pecan oil

SALAD

12 thin slices prosciutto
3 ounces crumbled goat cheese
2 tablespoons roasted pecans
20 to 24 sunflower sprouts
Fresh chive sprouts, for garnish

In a saucepan over medium-high heat, bring the vinegar to a boil. Lower heat and simmer until vinegar is reduced to a syrupy consistency. Remove from heat and slowly whisk in the pecan oil.

Using a ring mold, drape the prosciutto halfway over the mold's side. In the center, place half of the pecans, the crumbled goat cheese, and several sunflower sprouts. Dress with 1 tablespoon of dressing

Fold prosciutto over on top to form a pouch.

Arrange the remaining sprouts around the plate in a circle.

Finish with sprinkling pecans on the plate and another tbs. of dressing

Top with fresh chive sprouts.

*Serves 2*

### Sautéed Shrimp and Pattypan Squash in Parsley, Lemon, and Garlic Butter

2 tablespoons olive oil
10 fresh jumbo shrimp, peeled and deveined
Salt and freshly ground white pepper
8 pattypan squash, cut in quarters
1 shallot, chopped fine
2 cloves of garlic, chopped fine
Juice of ¹/₂ lemon
¹/₂ cup white wine
3 tablespoons unsalted butter
2 tablespoons chopped parsley

In a medium-size sauté pan, heat the olive oil and toss in the shrimp. Salt and pepper to taste and cook for 30 seconds on each side. Remove from the pan.

Add the squash to the pan and cook for 1 to 2 minutes, depending on their size. Add the chopped shallots and garlic to the squash. Cook another 20 seconds without browning. Remove vegetables from the pan.

Deglaze with the 1/2-cup of white wine and reduce by half. Remove pan from the heat and slowly whip in the butter and parsley.

Add the shrimp and vegetables back to the pan and finish cooking for 30 seconds.

Serve immediately.

*Serves 2*

*Bob Waggoner, a California native, has served as chef at fine restaurants across the United States, as well as in France and Venezuela. In 1988 he became the first American to own his own restaurant in France, the much-acclaimed Le Monte Cristo. He has appeared on many radio and television shows featuring his menus that combine unusual ingredients with classic techniques.*

# Michel Richard, Citronelle (Washington, D.C.)

## *St. Tropez-Santa Fe Black Bean Soup with Basil Puree*

1¹/₂ cups dried black beans, picked over and rinsed
12 cups water, plus more to soak the beans
1 large onion, peeled and diced
6 cloves garlic, peeled and minced
Salt and freshly ground black pepper to taste
¹/₃ cup olive oil
4 large cloves garlic, peeled
1¹/₂ cups (about 1¹/₂ ounces) fresh basil leaves
6 ounces green beans, ends snapped and strung, and
    sliced diagonally into 1-inch pieces (about 1¹/₂
    cups
2 small (about 8 ounces) zucchini, trimmed and
    cut into ¹/₂-inch dice
8 large fresh basil leaves, julienned, for garnish

Place the beans in a large pot and add enough water to cover them, plus about two inches more. Cover and set aside to soak at room temperature overnight.

Drain the beans and return them to the pot. Add 12 cups of water. Add the onion and garlic and bring to a boil, skimming off any foam. Reduce heat and simmer until the beans are very tender, about 2¹/₂ hours, stirring occasionally. Add water if needed, or boil the soup down until it is thickened to the consistency of minestrone. Season with salt and pepper.

Meanwhile, place the oil, garlic and basil in a blender. Puree until the mixture is smooth, pulsing on and off and stopping to scrape down the sides of the container. Season with salt and pepper.

Line a rack with paper towels. Cook the green beans for 3 minutes in a large pot of boiling water. Add the zucchini and cook until the beans are tender, for about 2 more minutes. Drain and rinse the vegetables under cold water and place them on the rack. Season with salt and pepper

To serve, return the soup to a boil. Stir $3/4$ of the vegetables and all of the puree into the soup. Ladle into 4 soup plates. Divide the remaining vegetables over the top of each soup. Garnish with basil julienne.

*Serves 4*

*In 2002, Michel Richard and Citronelle were awarded a double prize at the Capital Restaurant and Hospitality Awards. Richard was voted Chef of the Year and Citronelle was chosen as Best Fine Dining Restaurant, a double victory never awarded before.*

## Tory McPhail, Commander's Palace
## (New Orleans, Louisiana)

### *Veal Chop Tchoupitoulas*

3 quarts veal stock
$^1/_3$ cup vinegar
$^1/_3$ cup honey
1 tablespoon green peppercorns (fresh packed in
    brine), rinsed
1 roasted red bell pepper, cut in small dice
Kosher salt and freshly ground black pepper to taste
1 tablespoon butter
6 veal chops, each about 12 to 14 ounces and $1^1/_4$ to
    $1^1/_2$ inches thick
Your favorite Creole meat seasoning to taste
2 tablespoons vegetable oil

Bring the veal stock barely to a boil in a large pot
over high heat. Skim away any impurities that
might float to the top. Reduce the heat and barely
simmer to reduce sauce. Skim occasionally and
cook to a saucelike consistency, about $1^1/_4$ hours
to $2^1/_4$ hours. You'll be left with 1 to 2 cups. Strain
through a fine sieve and set aside.

Combine the vinegar and honey in a small
saucepan; stirring, bring to a boil over high heat,
then simmer for 10 to 15 minutes, until mixture
is reduced by about half. Add the reduced stock,
bring to a boil, and skim if necessary. Reduce the

heat and simmer until the sauce coats the back of a spoon, about 10 to 15 minutes. Add the green peppercorns and diced red pepper, season with salt and black pepper, and stir in the butter. Set aside and keep warm.

Bring the veal chops to room temperature. Place a large cast-iron skillet over high heat. Season the chops generously with meat seasoning. Place half the oil in the pan, bring to the smoking point, about 2 to 3 minutes, and place three chops in the pan. Cook 4 to 5 minutes, until the chops are golden brown. If the chops cook too fast, reduce heat. Turn the chops and cook 4 to 5 more minutes, which will bring them to medium rare. (Cook chops of this thickness for $3^1/2$ to 4 minutes per side for rare, 4 to 5 minutes for medium rare, 6 to 7 minutes for medium, 8 to 9 minutes for medium well, and 10 minutes for well done.) Keep warm. Add the remaining oil to the pan and cook the remaining chops. Serve with a bit of sauce over each chop.

When you make a reduction sauce, such as the one in this recipe, never let the stock boil. Reduce slowly and always skim away any impurities that float to the top. Depending on the stock, your reducing time and yield will vary Don't over reduce. A sauce that's too thick will become bitter.

Season at the end, not the beginning. Peppercorns will make the sauce spicy. As the sauce reduces, salt is more prevalent. Rinse the brine off the green peppercorns before adding them to the sauce. This sauce can keep for about 10 days in the refrigerator.

Professional cooks learn to associate feel and doneness. If you press a finger into medium-rare meat, it will spring back a bit. The longer the meat has cooked, the firmer its feel will be.

Chops are especially good cooked on a grill or under a broiler.

*Serves 6*

*Since 1880, Commander's Palace has been a New Orleans landmark known for its award-winning food quality and service. Brimming with the Brennan family's gracious Crescent City hospitality, Commander's Palace excels at making dining a special event. Commander's Palace was ranked New Orleans' most popular dining destination for a record fifteenth straight year in the 2002 Zagat survey and was chosen by the James Beard Foundation for the Outstanding Restaurant Award.*

### Jesse Cool, Flea St. Café
### (Menlo Park, California)

*Roast Ginger Pork with Mashed Ginger Yams,*
*Just-Warmed Tomatoes, Olives, and Capers*

2 pounds country pork chops
salt and pepper
10 cloves garlic, chopped
$1/4$ cup grated ginger
$1^1/2$ pounds seeded chopped tomatoes
$1/4$ cup extra virgin olive oil
$1/2$ cup seeded, chopped kalamata olives
3 tablespoons capers
$1/4$ cup ruby port
salt and pepper to taste

Preheat oven to 500° F.

Place the chops in a medium bowl and toss them with $2/3$ of the garlic, the ginger, and plenty of salt and pepper. Arrange on a heavy baking sheet and bake for about 1 hour.

Reduce heat to 375° F and roast for another hour or until the meat is very brown and crispy. Place on a large serving platter.

Meanwhile, gather the remaining ingredients. When the pork is cooked, place a 2 quart sauce pan sauté pan over medium heat and add the olive oil and remaining garlic and cook for one minute.

Add the olives, capers, chopped tomatoes, and port. Simmer for about 5 minutes.

Pour the sauce over the pork.

*Serves 4*

## Mashed Ginger Yams

1 1/2 pounds yams
1/8 cup grated ginger
2 ounces butter
2 teaspoons chopped fresh thyme
1 cup buttermilk
salt and pepper to taste

Peel, cook and mash yams. Add remaining ingredients. Season with salt and pepper.

*Serves 4*

*Jesse Cool started in the restaurant business thirty years ago with her innovative organic restaurant Late for the Train. Her passionate commitment to organics, sustainable practices, and caring for family and community are evidenced in her dedicated staff and through her restaurants, publications, and initiatives. Jesse Cool has been awarded the Menlo Park Environmental Award in 2001 and the NAWBO Top 100 Women Business Owners in 2002.*

## Tom Douglas, Dahlia Lounge, Etta's Seafood, and Palace Kitchen (Seattle, Washington)

### *Tom's Tasty Sashimi Tuna Salad with Whole Wheat Green Onion Pancakes*

The success of this dish depends on the quality of the tuna. Be sure it is fresh from a purveyor you trust, and one with a high turnover of fish. If you're buying from a Japanese market, ask for sashimi-grade tuna, the best available. Use the tuna immediately or store it in the refrigerator wrapped tightly in plastic on a tray of ice for up to a day.

12 ounces sashimi-grade tuna
1/3 cup sliced-on-bias green onions
1 2 1/2 ounce package kiware radish sprouts (or 1/3 cup fresh bean sprouts)
1/3 cup loosely packed fresh cilantro leaves
2 teaspoons toasted sesame seeds
9 tablespoons Sake Sauce, chilled (recipe below)
4 teaspoons peanut oil
1 teaspoon sesame oil
1/2 teaspoon chili oil
Green Onion Pancakes (recipe below)

Slice the tuna into strips about 1/8-inch thick. Place the sliced tuna in a bowl with the green onions, half the sprouts, cilantro, and sesame seeds. Add the Sake Sauce. The sauce must be cold, so as not to cook the raw tuna. Toss gently. Drizzle with the peanut, sesame, and chili oils and toss gently again. This salad is best served right away; it is not something you want to marinate for long because this will "cook" the fish.

Place equal amounts of the tuna salad on each of 4 plates. Drizzle extra dressing from the bowl around the plates. Cut each warm green onion pancake into 6 wedges and divide them among the plates. Garnish with the remaining sprouts. You can also add a lime wedge, wasabe tobiko or wasabe, and pickled ginger.

*Serves 4*

### Sake Sauce

$^1/_2$ cup sake
$^1/_4$ cup soy sauce
$^1/_4$ cup rice wine vinegar
1 small serrano chili, seeded and finely chopped
$^1/_4$ teaspoon minced garlic
1 tablespoon finely chopped green onion

Mix in a small bowl and let sit 20 minutes or more.

*Yields 1 cup*

### *Whole Wheat Green Onion Pancakes*

(The uncooked green onion pancakes will hold a day in the refrigerator wrapped well in plastic. Or you could fry them ahead, keep them at room temperature, and reheat them in a 350° oven for 5 minutes.)

1 large egg
2 teaspoons sesame oil
4 eight-inch whole wheat tortillas
2 teaspoons toasted sesame seeds
1/3 cup finely chopped green onions
1 tablespoon vegetable oil, or more as needed

In a small bowl, lightly beat the egg with the sesame oil. Brush each tortilla with the egg mixture and then sprinkle two of the tortillas with the scallions and sesame seeds. Sandwich the tortillas together, pressing down to seal. Heat 1 tablespoon of the vegetable oil in a sauté pan over medium heat. Add a pancake to the pan and cook until lightly browned on both sides, about 2 minutes per side. Repeat with remaining pancake. Keep warm until serving.

*Yields 2 pancakes*

*Tom Douglas has received numerous accolades, including the James Beard Award for Best North-*

*west Chef in 1994, and Best American Cookbook 2000 (for Tom Douglas's Seattle Kitchen). Starting with the acclaimed Café Sport in 1984, Douglas has helped to define the Northwest style known as Pacific Rim cuisine. His first restaurant was Dahlia Lounge, followed by Etta's Seafood and Palace Kitchen, which in 1997 was nominated for Best New Restaurant by the James Beard Foundation. Tom Douglas recently introduced a specialty foods line.*

### Sheri Davis, Dish (Atlanta, Georgia)

#### *Cool Cucumber Soup*

$1/2$ red onion, minced fine
Sea salt and freshly ground white pepper, to taste
1 pound lemon cucumbers (or any type of
    cucumber), diced
2 pounds organic cucumbers, peeled and with ends
    cut off
$1/4$ cup grapeseed oil
Juice of 1 lemon

Place the red onion in a large soup tureen and season with salt and white pepper. Add the diced lemon cucumber to the tureen. cucumber, add to the soup bain.

Pass the organic cucumbers through a juicer

and then transfer juice to a blender. Slowly blend in the grapeseed oil and lemon juice, making the cucumber juice frothy.

Add the blended juice and oil to the tureen; season to taste.

Serve this soup cold. For variety, serve this soup with grilled shrimp, crawfish-stuffed squash blossoms, salad burnet, or salmon croquettes.

*Serves 4*

### Sauteed Snapper with Asian Vegetables and Sesame Vinaigrette

2 cups water
1/4 cup julienned ginger
4 teaspoons olive oil, divided
4 (6-ounce) pieces snapper
salt and pepper to taste
2 cups shiitake mushrooms
6 heads baby bok choy
1 cup shredded daikon or radish
Sesame Vinaigrette (recipe below)

Add the water and the ginger to a small saucepan and bring to a boil.

Meanwhile, in a large saute pan, heat 2 teaspoons of olive oil. Season the snapper with salt and pepper, and add to the pan, searing it. Allow to cook for 2 minutes, then turn over and allow to cook for 2 more minutes. Remove from pan and keep warm.

Add remaining 2 teaspoons of olive oil to the pan; saute the shiitake mushrooms until tender. Toss them and add the bok choy and daikon. Using a slotted spoon, remove the ginger from the boiling water and add to the pan, along with 1/4 cup of the ginger water, allowing the water to steam the bok choy.

To serve, divide the vegetables among 4 plates; drizzle vegetables with Sesame Vinaigrette, and place one piece of snapper on top of the vegetables.

*Serves 4*

### Sesame Vinaigrette

1 cup water
1/4 cup soy sauce
3 tblsp sweet soy sauce
1 ounce toasted sesame seeds
2 tblsp sherry vinegar

Whisk together all ingredients.

*Yields 1 1/2 cups*

## Seared Thyme-Crusted Ahi Tuna with Seaweed and Sweet Chili

1/4 cup soy sauce
3 tablespoons sweet soy sauce
3 tablespoons sherry vinegar
4 tablespoons olive oil, divided, plus extra for
    seasoning fish
1 minced shallot
1 tablespoon minced fresh ginger
8 ounces fresh ahi tuna loin
1/4 cup fresh thyme
1/4 cup sweet chili garlic sauce
1 cup seaweed salad

In a small bowl, combine the soy sauces, vinegar, 3 tablespoons of olive oil, shallot, and ginger. Set aside.

Heat a cast-iron skillet over high heat.

While the pan is heating, season the tuna with salt and pepper. Rub the fish with a little olive oil and coat it with the thyme.

When the pan is very hot, add 1 tablespoon of olive oil and the fish. Using tongs, turn the tuna to sear it on all sides, leaving the inside very rare.

Remove the tuna from the heat and slice thin.

To serve, place 1 tablespoon of sweet chili garlic sauce in the center of each of 4 plates and top each with 1/4 cup of seaweed salad. Arrange the sliced tuna on each plate around the seaweed salad. Drizzle the soy sauce mixture on top.

*Serves 4 as an appetizer*

*Sheri Davis started her career in Milwaukee, Wisconsin at the James Beard Award–winning restaurant Sanford. After stints at the Quilted Giraffe and Le Bernadin in New York City, she moved to Atlanta where she held top positions at Brasserie Le Coze and Harvest. She then partnered with Bryan Wilson to open Dish in Atlanta, Georgia, which has won numerous awards and accolades in* Bon Appetit, Atlanta *magazine,* Zagat's, *and many other publications*

## Dominic Galati, Dominic's
### (St. Louis, Missouri)

### *Petti Di Pollo Alla Gina*
### *Chicken Breast Alla Gina*

4 boneless, skinless chicken breasts, sliced into
   cutlets and pounded thin
$1/2$ cup whole wheat flour
Salt and pepper to taste
3 tablespoons butter
3 tablespoons virgin olive oil
3 ounces Fontina cheese, shredded
3 ounces of prosciutto, diced

4 tablespoons tomato sauce
4 tablespoon chicken stock
4 tablespoons dry white wine
1 tablespoon chopped parsley, for garnish

Preheat the oven to 325° F.

Lightly coat the chicken slices with the flour and season with salt and pepper.

Melt the butter and olive oil together in a large oven-safe skillet over low heat; add the chicken slices and and lightly brown them. Top each one with a light layer of cheese and prosciutto. To the pan, add the tomato sauce, chicken stock, and wine, and heat gently.

Transfer the pan to the oven and heat until the cheese has melted and the sauce has slightly thickened. Serve on a heated serving plate covered with sauce and garnished with chopped parsley. Suggestions for accompaniments include green peas, mushrooms, or asparagus.

*Serves 4*

*Originally from Sicily, Dominic Galati started at the bottom and worked his way up in the restaurant business. He and his wife Jackie opened Dominic's in 1971 serving continental Italian cuisine with an emphasis on traditional regional dishes. Among the awards and honors Dominic's has received over the years are the 2001 Restau-*

*rant Hall of Fame Award, the DiRona Award (every year since 1977), an AAA Four Diamonds rating, and a 1999 International Award of Excellence. Dominic's was also voted one of the best two Italian restaurants in the country by the readers of* Conde Nast Traveler.

## Tom Rapp, Etats Unis (New York City)

### *Jorge's Vegetable Sauce for Fish*

1 red bell pepper
1 small eggplant, skinned and cut into large dice
Olive oil
Salt and pepper to taste
2 (6- to 8-ounce) fillets of fish (such as halibut, snapper, or swordfish)
1 medium yellow onion, peeled and chopped into 1-inch pieces
2 large cloves of garlic, peeled and coarsly chopped
1/4 cup chopped parsley
1/4 cup whole fresh basil leaves
Juice of 1/2 lemon

Preheat oven to 400°F.

Lightly oil the bell pepper and the eggplant pieces; place on an oiled cookie sheet and roast the pepper for ten minutes until the skin is lightly browned, and the eggplant until it is cooked through, turning the eggplant once. Remove from oven and, when cool, gently remove skin, stem, and seeds from the pepper and chop into $1/2$-inch by 1-inch pieces. Place the pepper and eggplant in a medium bowl.

Lightly oil, salt, and pepper the fish and place on a small, shallow, oven-proof dish lined with aluminum foil. Roast uncovered for approximately 12 to 15 minutes, depending on thickness of fish.

Meanwhile, sauté the onion in olive oil until it is soft but not browned. Place in the bowl with the pepper. In the same pan, brown the garlic; add the parsley and whole basil leaves and saute until the herbs are wilted. Add to the pepper, eggplant, and onion mixture. Salt and pepper the vegetables to taste and add additional olive oil and the lemon juice.

To serve, center each piece of fish on a plate and spoon the vegetables over it. Sliced ripe avocado with cherry tomatoes tossed in a light red-wine vinaigrette make a nice accompaniment.

*Serves 2*

*Tom Rapp received degrees in art history and architecture. Cooking became a passionate hobby when he "discovered" Julia Child in 1963. He opened his first restaurant Etats-Unis in 1992 with his son Jonathan. Etats-Unis has received national recognition and acclaim for its intimate style and a menu that changes nightly.*

# Francis Perrin, Frederick's Restaurant
# (San Antonio, Texas)

## *Filet Mignon with Green Peppercorn Sauce and Wild Mushroom Flan*

### WILD MUSHROOM FLAN

1 teaspoon clarified butter
$1/2$ teaspoon minced garlic
1 ounce shiitake mushrooms, diced
1 ounce chanterelle mushrooms, diced
1 ounce button mushrooms, diced
2 tablespoons white wine
3 eggs
2 cups heavy cream

### GREEN PEPPERCORN SAUCE

1 tablespoon green peppercorns
1 ounce cognac
1 ounce Port
1 ounce Madeira
3 ounces cabernet wine
5 ounces veal stock

5 (8-ounce) center-cut beef tenderloins
salt and pepper

Preheat the oven to 350°F. Preheat a grill or broiler for the tenderloin.

Prepare the flan: Heat a medium skillet over medium heat. Add the clarified butter, and sauté the garlic in the butter for 30 seconds. Add the mushrooms and sauté for 2 minutes more. Add the white wine and allow the mixture to reduce until the mixture is just moist. Remove from heat.

In a medium bowl, beat the eggs with the cream. Add the mushrooms and mix well.

Spray 5 three-ounce cups with nonstick spray and pour the mixture into each one of them. Place cups in a bain-marie and bake for 40 minutes.

Meanwhile, prepare the sauce: flambé the peppercorns with all the liquor and reduce to approximately 2 ounces. Add veal stock and bring to a boil. Set aside.

Salt and pepper the beef, and cook until medium rare.

*Serves 5*

### Butternut Squash Soup

1 butternut squash, peeled, seeded, and cubed
2 slices bacon, diced
1 small onion, chopped
$1/3$ cup diced carrot
2 quarts chicken stock
1 pinch nutmeg
1 pinch cinnamon
1 pint heavy cream
Salt and pepper to taste

In a large pot, sauté the bacon for 3 minutes, then add onion and carrots and sauté until bacon is slightly crispy. Add squash followed by chicken stock and all seasonings. Boil moderately for 45 minutes, then puree in a blender. Pour soup through a small strainer and return it to the stove. Add the cream, bring to boil, and add salt and pepper to taste.

*Serves 6*

*Chef Francis Perrin was born and raised in Switzerland, where at age 19 he went to culinary school in Neuchatel. In his early years Chef Perrin traveled through Europe working in some of the finest restaurants. In the late 1970s he came to Washington and worked at Rive Gauche, Tiberio and Jean Pierre. When Chef Perrin became friends with Frederick Costa the two came to San Antonio to open the popular E'Toile. Desiring to bring their two homelands together, they opened Frederick's in the summer of 2000. Chef Perrin's classic approach to elegant cuisine embraces the finest of Asian and French food.*

## Rick Bayless, Frontera Grill and Topolobampo (Chicago, Illinois)

### *Ceviche Clasico*

1 pound fresh, skinless snapper, bass, halibut or other ocean fish fillets, cut into 1/2-inch cubes or slightly smaller

About 1 1/2 cups fresh lime juice

1 medium white onion, chopped into 1/4-inch pieces

1 pound (2 medium-large round or 6 to 8 plum) ripe tomatoes, chopped into 1/4-inch pieces

Fresh hot green chiles to taste (roughly 2 to 3 serranos or 1 to 2 jalapeños), stemmed, seeded and finely chopped

1/3 cup chopped fresh cilantro, plus a few leaves for garnish

1/3 cup chopped pitted green olives (choose manzanillos for a typical Mexican flavor)

1 to 2 tablespoons olive oil, preferably extra-virgin (optional, but recommended to give a glistening appearance)

Salt

3 tablespoons fresh orange juice

1 large or 2 small ripe avocados, peeled, pitted and diced

Whole wheat tostadas, tortilla chips, or Triscuits® for serving

Marinate the fish: In a 1½-quart glass or stainless steel bowl, combine the fish, lime juice and onion. You'll need enough juice to cover the fish and allow it to float somewhat freely; too little juice means unevenly "cooked" fish. Cover and refrigerate for about 4 hours, until a cube of fish no longer looks raw when broken open. Pour into a colander and drain off the lime juice.

Mix the flavorings: In a large bowl, mix together the tomatoes, green chiles, cilantro, olives and optional olive oil. Stir in the fish, then taste and season with salt, usually about ¾ teaspoon, and the orange juice or sugar (the sweetness of the orange juice or sugar helps balance some of the typical tanginess of the ceviche) Cover and refrigerate if not serving immediately.

Serve the ceviche: Just before serving, stir in the diced avocado, being careful not to break up the pieces. For serving, you have several options: Set out your ceviche in a large bowl and let people spoon it onto individual plates to eat with chips; serve small bowls of ceviche (I like to lay a bed of frisée lettuce in each bowl before spooning in the ceviche) and serve whole-wheat tostadas, chips or whole wheat Triscuits,® alongside; or pile the ceviche onto chips or tostadas and pass around for guests to consume on these edible little plates. Whichever direction you choose, garnish the ceviche with leaves of cilantro before setting it center stage.

Working ahead: The fish can be marinated a day in advance; after about 4 hours, when the fish is "cooked," drain it so that it won't become too limy. For the freshest flavor, add the flavorings to the fish no more than a couple of hours before serving.

*Serves 8 as an appetizer, 12 as a nibble*

### Mexican Beans

FOR THE BROTHY BEANS

1 pound (about 2¹/₂ cups) dried beans (any color you wish, from black to red, tan, white or speckled)

2 tablespoons rich-tasting pork lard (or even bacon drippings or fat rendered from chorizo sausage) or vegetable oil

1 medium white onion, chopped

1 large sprig fresh epazote (optional but delicious—especially with black beans)

Salt

FOR TURNING BROTHY BEANS INTO REFRITOS

¹/₄ cup vegetable oil or rich-tasting pork lard (or one of the other options listed above)

1 medium white onion, chopped

4 large garlic cloves, peeled and finely chopped

About ³/₄ cup (3 ounces) crumbled Mexican queso fresco or other crumbly fresh cheese, such as salted pressed farmer's cheese or feta, for garnish

Prepare the simple boiled beans (frijoles de la olla): Though beans in the United States are sold very clean, it's always a good idea to pour them out onto a baking sheet and sort through them, removing any little stones or debris you encounter; scoop the beans into a colander and rinse.

Pour the beans into a deep medium-large (4- to 6-quart) pot (preferably a heavy Dutch oven or Mexican earthenware olla). Measure in 2 1/2 quarts water, then remove any beans that float (they're ones that are not fully formed). Add the fat or oil, onion and the optional epazote. Bring to a strong rolling boil, then reduce the heat (low to medium-low on most stoves) to keep the liquid at a very gentle simmer—any more than a slight rolling movement will cause the beans to break up some during cooking. Set a cover slightly askew (no need to cover the narrow-mouthed Mexican olla—its design takes care of maintaining even heat and controlling evaporation) and gently simmer, adding water as needed to keep the liquid level roughly the same, until the beans are thoroughly tender, about 2 hours.

Stir in 1 1/2 teaspoons salt and simmer for 15 minutes longer to allow the salt to be absorbed, then taste and season with additional salt if you think necessary. The beans are now ready to serve in small bowls or to mash and fry.

Prepare the frijoles refritos: Pour the beans into

a colander set over a large bowl; discard the epazote if you used it. In a large (12-inch) heavy skillet (preferably nonstick), heat the oil or other fat over medium. Add the onion and cook, stirring regularly, until deeply golden brown, 7 to 8 minutes. Add the garlic and cook until very fragrant, about 1 minute. Now, begin adding the beans to the skillet a couple of large spoonfuls at a time, mashing them to a coarse puree with a wooden bean masher, an old-fashioned potato masher or the back of a large spoon. When all the beans have been added, stir in enough bean broth to give the mixture the consistency of soft mashed potatoes—this not-so-rich version of frijoles refritos will thicken as it continues cooking and especially as it cools at the table.

Taste the beans and season with additional salt if necessary. Scoop onto a serving platter or spoon onto individual plates, sprinkle with the crumbled cheese and stud with the optional tortilla chips. You're ready to serve.

Working ahead: Beans, whether simply boiled or fried luxuriously in lard, will keep for 4 or 5 days in the refrigerator, tightly covered. The texture and flavor of the boiled beans' broth will improve after a day or so.

*Makes 7 to 8 cups whole brothy beans or 5 cups fried beans, serving 8 to 10*

## Grilled Salmon with Lemon-and-Thyme-Scented Salsa Veracruzana

1/4 cup olive oil, preferably extra-virgin, plus a little
   for oiling the salmon
1 medium white onion, thinly sliced
4 garlic cloves, peeled and finely chopped
3 pounds (6 medium-large round or 18 to 24 plum)
   ripe tomatoes (you might want to use a mixture
   of yellow and red tomatoes), cored and chopped
   into 1/2-inch pieces (about 7 cups)
2 tablespoons chopped fresh thyme (lemon thyme
   is wonderful here, if that's an option), plus a few
   sprigs for garnish
2 teaspoons finely chopped lemon zest (colored rind
   only—no white pith)
1 cup pitted, roughly sliced green olives, preferably
   manzanillo olives
1/4 cup capers, drained and rinsed
3 pickled jalapeño chiles, stemmed, seeded and
   thinly sliced
Salt
Six 7- to 8-ounce salmon steaks, about 1 inch thick

Prepare the sauce: In a medium (4- or 5-quart)
pot (preferably a Dutch oven or Mexican cazuela),
heat the olive oil over medium. Add the onion
and cook, stirring regularly, until just beginning
to brown, about 5 minutes. Add the garlic and
cook 1 minute more, stirring several times. Raise

the heat to medium-high and add the tomatoes, thyme, lemon zest and half of the olives, capers and chiles. Simmer briskly, stirring frequently, for about 5 minutes to evaporate some of the liquid. Reduce the heat to medium-low, stir in 1 cup of water and simmer for 15 minutes. Taste and season with salt, usually about 1 teaspoon. Remove from the heat to cool.

Grill the fish: Heat a gas grill to medium-high or light a charcoal fire and let it burn just until the coals are covered with gray ash and very hot. Reduce the heat on one side of the gas grill to medium-low or set up the charcoal grill for indirect cooking by banking all the coals to one side, leaving the other half of the grill empty. Set the cooking grate in place, cover the grill and let the grate heat up, 5 minutes or so.

If desired, use a wooden pick to skewer the ends of each salmon steak together so they don't tear off during the grilling. Brush or spray both sides of the salmon steaks with oil and sprinkle with salt. Lay the salmon steaks over the hottest part of the fire and cook for about 4 minutes, until nicely browned underneath. Using a spatula, carefully flip the fish over onto the cooler side of the grill for 2 to 4 minutes to get the salmon to that medium-rare, still-slightly-translucent-in-the-center stage that I love. (Or judge your own preference for doneness accordingly.)

Cool the fish in the sauce: Spoon the sauce into

a deep platter and nestle the fish in it. Let stand at room temperature for about an hour to bring to-gether the flavors of fish and sauce.

To serve, sprinkle the fish with the remaining olives, capers, and chiles and decorate with thyme sprigs, and you're ready to serve.

Working ahead: Everything about this dish says "make ahead." The sauce will keep for several days in the refrigerator, well covered. In fact, the whole dish can be made a day ahead without much compromise in quality—simply wrap it and refrigerate. Let the fish and sauce warm to room temperature before serving. If you make the dish early on the day you're serving, don't let it stand at room temperature any longer than 2 hours without refrigeration.

*Serves 6*

*Rick Bayless has won our nation's highest chef honor: the James Beard Foundation's National Chef of the Year. He's also won the Julia Child/ IACP Cookbook of the Year award for* Rick Bay-less's Mexican Kitchen. *His other cookbooks in-clude* Authentic Mexican, Salsas That Cook *and* Rick Bayless's Mexico: One Plate at a Time. *His famed Chicago restaurants, Frontera Grill and Topolobampo, have both won many awards, in-cluding the coveted Ivy Award. Bayless also hosts PBS's* Mexico: One Plate at a Time.

## Galatoire's (New Orleans, Louisiana)

### *Crabmeat Sardou*

8 artichokes
1 pound jumbo lump crabmeat
2 tablespoons clarified butter
1 cup Creamed Spinach (recipe below)
1 cup Hollandaise Sauce (recipe below)
2 pinches paprika, for garnish

Place the artichokes into a medium-sized pot filled with enough water to cover. Cover and boil for 30 minutes over medium heat. Drain and cool. Peel the leaves from the artichokes and discard. Remove the hearts and, using a spoon, remove and discard the choke. Slice off the remaining portion of the stems from the bottoms.

Sauté the crabmeat in the clarified butter over medium heat. Remove from heat and drain off excess butter.

Arrange four serving plates, spoon equal portions of Creamed Spinach onto each, then lay 2 artichoke bottoms over each spinach bed. Spoon equal portions of crabmeat over the bottoms, then top with a spoonful of Hollandaise Sauce. Garnish with a light sprinkle of paprika.

*Serves 4*

## *Creamed Spinach*

4 cups milk
$^1/_2$ teaspoon salt
$^1/_2$ teaspoon white pepper
Pinch cayenne pepper
1 bay leaf
$^1/_2$ cup white wine
$^1/_2$ cup butter
$^1/_2$ cup flour
1 cup heavy cream, reserved (if needed)
3 cups fresh cooked spinach
Salt to taste
$^1/_8$ teaspoon white pepper
1 chopped hard-boiled egg

In a small pot, heat the milk to a simmer, Reduce heat and add salt, pepper, cauenne, bay leaf and the white wine. Simmer for a few minutes. In a separate large pot, melt the butter over low heat and add the flour to make a roux, constantly stirring with a wire whisk. Strain the milk through a fine sieve and pour it into the roux pot, stirring constantly in a circular motion. The sauce will thicken. Add heavy cream, if needed, to enrich the sauce or to thin it out if it becomes too thick . Allow to simmer for 5 minutes more to cook the flour taste out.

Over medium-low heat, fold the spinach into the sauce. Add salt and pepper and simmer for

15 minutes, stirring with a wooden spoon. Add chopped hard-boiled egg, then stir. Remove from heat and keep warm until ready to serve.

### Hollandaise Sauce

6 egg yolks
2 tablespoons solid butter, cut into small pieces
Pinch salt
Pinch cayenne pepper
1 teaspoon lemon juice
1 teaspoon red wine vinegar
2 tablespoons cold water
2 cups clarified butter

In a bain-marie or double boiler, combine the egg yolks with the 2 tablespoons of solid butter, calt, cayenne, lemon juice, and red wine vinegar. Using a wire whisk, slowly blend the mixture over medium heat, allowing the butter to melt into the mixture. Continue to whisk until the mixture takes on a thick, almost coarse texture.

Remove from heat and add the water. This will cool the mixture and prevent curdling.

Using a ladle, slowly pour in the clarified butter, whisking the mixture constantly with a circular motion. The sauce should achieve a nice, thick consistency.

Note: Do not refrigerate and keep at a constant

temperature. Any sudden change in temperature will cause the sauce to separate or break.

## Oysters Rockefeller

3 dozen large oysters
3 cups chopped spinach
1/2 cup finely chopped green onions
1/2 cup finely chopped yellow onions
2/3 cup finely chopped parsley
1 rib chopped celery
1 teaspoon minced garlic
Pinch ground thyme
Pinch ground anise
1/4 teaspoon salt
1/4 teaspoon white pepper
1/4 teaspoon black pepper
1 tablespoon red wine vinegar
1 teaspoon Worcestershire sauce
2 tablespoon herbsaint
1 cup clarified butter
1 cup fine whole grain bread crumbs
6 cups rock salt
6 lemon wedges

Preheat oven to 350°F.

Place oysters in a small pot and add water to cover. Simmer for 5 minutes over medium-high heat. Drain and set aside.

To make the Rockefeller sauce, in a food

processor combine the spinach, green onions, yellow onions, parsley, celery, garlic, thyme, anise, salt, white pepper, black pepper, red wine vinegar, Worcestershire, herbsaint, and butter. Coarsely puree the above ingredients. Transfer to a mixing bowl, then fold in bread crumbs, blending well.

Fill six 8-inch cake pans with rock salt to cover bottoms. Arrange 6 oyster half-shells in each. Place one oyster in each shell. Fill a pastry bag with Rockefeller sauce. Pipe equal portions of sauce over each shell. Place in the oven and bake for 25 minutes.

Remove and transfer pans to napkin-covered serving plates. Garnish with lemon wedges.

*Serves 6*

*Since 1905, diners have raised their glasses to toast the good life at Galatoire's, an elegant New Orleans dining haven steeped in tradition. The timeless ambience mirrors the superlative French Creole cuisine.*

*The extensive menu reads like a catalogue of ageless New Orleans favorites: shrimp remoulade, oysters Rockefeller, Creole gumbo, crabmeat Maison, shrimp Clemenceau, pompano with sautéed crabmeat meuniere, and banana bread pudding.*

*Galatoire's was named as one of the nation's Top 50 restaurants in the October, 2001 issue of*

Gourmet *magazine, and has garnered many other awards during its ninety-seven-year history. Considered the grande dame of New Orleans' old-line restaurants, tradition has been maintained with little change through the decades.*

## Daniel Orr, Guastavino's (New York City)

### *Herb-Perfumed Chicken Breast with Vegetable Fleurettes and Sweet Potatoes*

1 (12- to 16-ounce) skinless, boneless chicken
   breast
1 teaspoon Master Blend (recipe below)
$1/2$ cup chopped mixed herbs such as basil, chervil,
   chives, tarragon, and parsley
1 small clove garlic, chopped
5 drops hot pepper sauce such as Tabasco
$1/2$ teaspoon sea salt, divided
10 turns of a pepper mill
2 small sweet potatoes, peeled and cut into
   5 pieces each
10 cauliflower fleurettes
10 broccoli fleurettes
10 cherry tomatoes
1 tablespoon lemon juice
1 tablespoon olive oil
10 basil leaves, cut into chiffonade
Herb sprigs for garnish

This is a real no-brainer for those evenings when you want something simple, fresh, and clean-tasting.

Cut the chicken breast in half and make five diagonal slits in each half.

In a small bowl combine the Master Blend, herbs, garlic, hot pepper sauce, $1/4$ teaspoon sea salt and 5 turns of the pepper mill. Stuff each slit in the chicken with a generous amount of this mixture.

Place the chicken and sweet potatoes in a medium-sized steamer. Steam for 6 minutes, then add the cauliflower and steam for 5 minutes. Add the broccoli to the steamer and steam for 3 to 4 minutes. Top the broccoli with the cherry tomatoes and steam just to heat through, 1 minute. Take care not to overcook the broccoli, or it will discolor.

In a medium-sized mixing bowl combine the lemon juice, oil, chiffonaded basil, and the remaining salt and pepper; mix well.

Remove the vegetables to the bowl with the dressing and gently toss to coat the vegetables; taste and adjust the seasoning as necessary and spoon onto a serving platter. Top with the chicken breasts and pour any remaining dressing over the chicken. Garnish with the herbs and serve at once.

*Serves 2*

## *Master Blend—New Regime*

This is great on everything. Add the blend to bacon during the last third of cooking; sautéed chicken livers, scallops, shrimp; roasts of all kinds; stuffing; pâtés and terrines; Persian rice; and slow-cooked green beans with tomatoes. Use it as a rub for poultry before roasting and in dredging flour for sautés.

2 tablespoons coriander
2 pieces star anise
1 tablespoon fennel seeds, half raw, half toasted
2 teaspoons mustard seeds
5 cardadorn seeds
1 teaspoon cumin seeds
1 teaspoon ginger powder
1 ($1/2$) stick cinnamon
1 teaspoon white peppercorns
1 teaspoon black peppercorns
3 dried bay leaves
$1/2$ teaspoon whole mace

Grind together finely in a spice grinder.

## *Tuna Steak aux Poivres*

1 pound tuna steak (1 to 1¹/₂ inches thick, dark part
  removed)
1 teaspoon salt
2 tablespoons Mixed Pepper Blend (recipe below)
1 tablespoon olive oil
1 medium onion, julienned
3 cloves garlic, sliced into thin rounds
4 cups thinly sliced vegetables such as yellow
  squash, baby bok choy, thin green beans, and red
  peppers
¹/₂ cup fish or chicken stock
¹/₂ cup chopped basil
2 basil tops for garnish

Season the tuna with the salt and Mixed Pepper
Blend.

Place a 2-quart, heavy-bottomed saucepan over
high heat. Add the oil and carefully place the tuna
in the center of the pan. Cook until well browned,
3 to 5 minutes, then turn the tuna to brown the
other side. Remove the tuna from the pan.

In the same pan place the onion, garlic, and
vegetables. Cook, stir-frying, for 3 to 5 minutes.
Add the stock and cook, covered, for 3 to 4 minutes until the vegetables are tender but still crisp.

Stir in the chopped basil, remove the pan from
the heat, and place the vegetables on a warm serv-

ing plate. Place the tuna on top and garnish with basil tops.

The cooking time depends on the thickness of the tuna. It is important not to overcook it or it will be dry. It should have the look and feel of beef cooked medium-rare.

Salmon and swordfish are good variations, but the swordfish must be cooked all the way through.

*Serves 2*


### Mixed Pepper Blend—Aux Poivres

Use to season roasted jumbo sea scallops; venison chops with juniper; seared spiced tuna fillet; and as a crust for New York sirloin steaks. Sprinkle on soups and salads for a peppery crunch.

Mix with Master Blend (above) and brown sugar for "oven barbecued" salmon fillets.

2 tablespoons cracked white pepper
2 tablespoons cracked black pepper
1 teaspoon crushed red pepper (cayenne)
3 tablespoons crushed fennel seeds
4 tablespoons crushed coriander seeds
2 tablespoons crushed Szechuan pepper
1 teaspoon crushed Guinea pepper

Blend the ingredients together thoroughly.

### Barley Salad with Chili, Herb, and Lime Vinaigrette

10 asparagus spears
1 yellow squash
3/4 cup barley
2 tablespoons olive oil
1 tablespoons cider vinegar
1/2 teaspoon chili powder
Juice of 1 lime
1 teaspoon diced lime zest
Juice of 1/2 lemon
Salt
Freshly ground pepper
1/4 cup diced sweet red pepper
1/4 cup diced yellow pepper

Blanch the asparagus spears in boiling water for 5 to 7 minutes; drain and chill. Cut off and reserve 3-inch tips and cut the stems into thin rounds.

Cut the yellow squash into small sticks, blanch briefly, drain, and chill.

Rinse the barley thoroughly under cold running water and drain. In a medium-sized saucepan cover the barley with 3 1/2 cups cold water. Bring to a boil, then reduce the heat to a simmer and cook for 35 to 45 minutes until the barley is tender and no longer raw, but is chewy to the bite. Rinse the barley under cold water and drain.

To make the vinaigrette, whisk together the

oil, 1 tablespoon water, the vinegar, chili powder, lime juice and zest, lemon juice, and salt and pepper to taste.

In a large bowl combine the chilled barley, asparagus rounds, squash, red and yellow peppers, and the vinaigrette; toss well and adjust the seasoning as necessary. Top with the asparagus tips. The salad will keep, tightly covered, in the refrigerator for 2 to 3 days.

Additional herbs and peppers can be added along with the asparagus tips just before serving. This salad is also wonderful in pita sandwiches or served with grilled fish or chicken.

*Serves 2*

*Chef Daniel Orr is executive chef at Guastavino's where he was awarded the Best New Restaurant in America award from* Esquire Magazine. *He has also cooked in restaurants throughout Europe and was executive chef at New York's famed La Grenouille.*

## Aaron L. Keller, Humpy's Alehouse (Anchorage, Alaska)

### Grilled Sea Scallops with Roasted Tomato Relish, Napa Cabbage, and Black Bean Ragout

2 cups dry black beans
6 cups water
6 cups vegetable stock
2 bay leaves
1 teaspoon chopped fresh thyme
1 small onion, chopped
2 cloves garlic, minced
1 shallot, minced
5 Roma tomatoes, divided (1 chopped, 4 quartered)
1 teaspoon cumin
1 teaspoon coriander
Pinch of cayenne pepper
Salt and white pepper to taste
1 leek, washed and julienned
2 oranges, segmented
6 tablespoons olive oil, divided
3 tablespoons balsamic vinegar
20 large sea scallops
1 head napa cabbage, quartered (or any type of
    cabbage or bok choy)
2 tablespoons fresh chopped basil, for garnish

Soak the black beans in 6 cups of water overnight.
   Drain beans and rinse well. In a large saucepan,

simmer the beans in the vegetable stock until the amount of liquid is reduced by half. Add the bay leaves, thyme, onion, garlic, shallot, chopped tomato, cumin, coriander, and cayenne. Continue to simmer until beans thicken and are tender. Season with salt and white pepper. *Note:* This step can be done a day in advance to let the flavors to develop; simply reheat beans before continuing with recipe.

Preheat oven to 400°F. Preheat a grill or broiler to 400°F.

Place the 4 quartered tomatoes, leeks, and orange segments in a large bowl; add 2 tablespoons of olive oil, balsamic vinegear, and salt and white pepper to taste and toss thoroughly to coat. Spread the mixture evenly on a baking pan and roast until golden brown (about 15 minutes). Remove from oven and allow to cool. When cabbage is cool, julienne it.

Meanwhile, brush the scallops and cabbage with 4 tablespoons of olive oil. Grill the cabbage on all sides until slightly tender. Set aside and keep warm. Grill the scallops for about two to three minutes per side, depending on their size. Avoid overcooking, as they will continue cooking for a few minutes when removed from the grill.

To serve, place 1/4 cup black beans in the center of each of four plates, heap some cabbage over the beans, and place five scallops on top of the cabbage on each plate. Spoon the tomato and orange mixture over the scallops and garnish with fresh basil.

*Serves 4*

*Beginning his career at the Anchorage Hilton as a chef's apprentice, Aaron Keller then spent a year at the Kona Hawaii Hilton. He has since held top positions at several Anchorage restaurants including the chef de cuisine spot at The Top of the World at the Anchorage Hilton. He is currently executive chef at Humpy's Alehouse in Anchorage.*

## Mark Abernathy, Loca Luna Bistro and Bene Vita Ristorante (Little Rock, Arkansas)

### Grilled Salmon Filets with Jalapeno Mustard Cream Sauce

6 salmon fillets
2 tablespoons vegetable oil
salt and pepper to taste
2 tablespoons unsalted butter
1 cup chopped red onion
1 tablespoon chopped canned jalapeños (rinse them under hot water before chopping)
2 large garlic cloves, minced
1/2 cup chicken stock
1 cup white wine

2 cups heavy cream or half-and-half
3 tablespoons stone-ground whole grain mustard
2 tablespoons finely chopped cilantro
Pinch nutmeg
Cilantro sprigs for garnish

Prepare a grill or preheat the broiler.

Coat the salmon fillets with the oil and salt and pepper to taste. Grill or broil salmon until done; do not overcook.

Meanwhile, prepare the sauce: In a medium saucepan over medium heat, melt the butter and saute the red onion, jalapeños, and garlic for 4 minutes. Raise the heat to hight and add the chicken stock and wine. Bring to a boil and allow mixture to reduce by two-thirds.

Add the heavy cream or half-and-half and return to a boil. Remove pan from the heat and stir in the mustard, cinaltro, nutmeg, and salt and pepper to taste. Strain the sauce and return it to the heat, stirring often, until the sauce reaches the desired thickness.

To serve, pool the sauce on each serving plate and place the salmon on the sauce. Garnish with cilantro.

*Serves 6*

### Tuscan White Bean Soup

5 whole tomatoes
1 canned chipotle chili in adobo sauce
2 tablespoons canola oil
1 large onion, chopped
2 cloves garlic, finely chopped
$1/2$ cup chopped celery
6 cups chicken broth
1 pound dried white beans
2 tablespoons chopped parsley
1 teaspoon salt
1 teaspoon white pepper
$1^1/2$ cups water

Preheat the broiler.

Core the tomatoes and roast them under the broiler until they start to blacken. Place the roasted tomatoes and the chipotle pepper in a blender and puree them.

In a 4-quart soup pot, heat the canola oil. Add the onion, garlic, and celery and saute until tender; add the pureed tomato mixture from the blender. Stir in the chicken broth and the beans, parsley, salt, and pepper.

Bring to a boil; boil for two minutes, and then reduce the heat, cover, and simmer for $1^1/4$ hours. Add $1^1/2$ cups of water to the soup; continue to simmer for another hour, or until the beans are tender.

Pour $1^1/2$ cups of soup into the blender and

process until smooth. Repeat with another 1¹/₂ cups
of soup; return to the pot and reheat.

This soup is great served with a grilled garlic
pork loin.

*Serves 6*

*Mark Abernathy is is a nationally recognized chef
and restaurateur and has been featured as one of
America's top chefs in such publications as* Bon
Appetit, Southern Living, Cook's, The New York
Times, Gourmet, Texas Monthly, The Washington Post, Atlanta Journal, Food Arts *and many
other fine publications. He is also the host and
creator of a syndicated cooking show called Today's Cuisine. In addition, he is a follower of the
Sugar Busters! lifestyle.*

### Chef Tim Love, The Lonesome Dove Western Bistro (Fort Worth, Texas)

*Double Cut Wild Boar Chop
With Grilled Okra*

1 gallon Salt Brine for Poultry or Pork (recipe below)
4 (12- to16-ounce) double-cut wild boar chops
  (domestic pork may be substituted)
1 pound fresh okra
¹/₄ cup Lonesome Dove Game Rub

olive oil
Kosher salt
Cracked black pepper

Heat brine to 100 degrees, place chops in brine, and refrigerate uncovered for 1 hour.

Preheat the oven to 375°F. Preheat a grill.

Remove chops from brine, and season lightly with salt and pepper. Then season heavily with Lonesome Dove Game Rub

Heat olive oil in a sauté pan and sear each chop for 2 minutes on each side. Place chops on a baking sheet and let stand for 10 minutes. Place chops on the baking sheet in the oven and bake for 10 minutes.

Meanwhile, season the okra with olive oil, salt, and pepper; grill for 2$^1$/$_2$ minutes, turning every 30 seconds.

Serve the chops and okra together as soon as the meat is done.

*Serves 4*

### *Lonesome Dove BBQ Game Rub*

This is good on just about anything except maybe your cereal in the morning.

1 cup guajillo chile powder
1 cup Kosher salt

$^1/_2$ cup cumin, ground
$^1/_4$ cup rosemary, finely chopped
$^1/_4$ cup thyme leaves, finely chopped
$^3/_4$ cup black pepper, coursely ground
$^1/_4$ cup garlic powder
$^1/_4$ cup brown sugar

Combine all ingredients, and mix well.

Put what you don't use in a separate container, and keep in your pantry.

### Salt Brine for Poultry or Pork

You can brine any poultry or pork product. Poultry tends to need 3 times the amount of time in the brine as pork does. Do not brine pork over 2 hours; it really absorbs salt very quickly. Remember, after pork has been properly brined, it does not need to be cooked medium well or better. The salt has already cured all the harmful bacteria and allows you to have a nice, moist pork product.

*Makes 1 gallon*

1 gallon water
$^1/_4$ cup red chile flakes
$^1/_2$ cup Kosher salt
1 bay leaf
2 garlic cloves

Add all ingredients in a stockpot and bring to a boil; boil until salt dissolves.

Allow the liquid to cool to 38° F or cooler. Add your meat and refrigerate.

Refrigerate 1 to 2 hours for pork products; 4 to 6 hours for poultry, depending on the size of the bird.

*Yields 1 gallon*

*Tim Love may have started cooking out of necessity as a college student, but he has built his twelve-year career based on his passion for good food, friends, and wine. He is the owner and executive chef of the Lonesome Dove Western Bistro in the Fort Worth Stockyards National Historic District. He also owns a consulting firm for fine dining establishments and teaches cooking classes around the nation. Tim has created his own private label wines, as well as his own line of gourmet sauces available at specialty markets.*

# Deborah Knight, Mosaic (Scottsdale, Arizona)

## *Seasonal Fish en Papillote*

3 cups boiling water
1 1/2 cup sundried tomatoes (not oil-packed)
4 medium garlic cloves
1 medium shallot, peeled
1/3 cup olive oil
3/4 cup chicken or vegetable stock
4 1/2 teaspoons chopped parsley, divided
2 1/2 teaspoons chopped thyme, divided
2 1/2 teaspoons chopped oregano, divided
2 1/2 teaspoons chopped chives, divided
Juice of 1 lemon, divided
1/8 teaspoon salt
1/8 teaspoon pepper
4 tablespoon white wine
4 tablespoon chicken stock
1 celery stalk, julienned
1/2 onion, julienned
4 tablespoons quartered picholine or other green
   olive
4 fillets fish such as salmon, sea bass, or cod
salt and white pepper to taste

4 sheets baking paper cut into large heart shapes (or
   premade aluminum-foil pockets)

Preheat the oven to 400°F.

Reconstitute sundried tomatoes in 3 cups boiling water (let sit about 5 minutes). Drain and squeeze out excess water.

Mince the garlic and shallots in a food processor. Add the sundried tomatoes and continue to process. Add the olive oil and stock. Continue to process until the mixture is a paste, about 45 seconds. Add 3 teaspoons parsley, 1 teaspoon thyme, 1 teaspoon oregano, 1 teaspoon chives, juice of 1/2 lemon, salt, and pepper. Process once more and set aside.

In a bowl, combine white wine, juice of 1/2 lemon, and chicken stock. In another bowl combine the celery, onion, and picholine or olives. In a third, small bowl, combine 1 1/2 teaspoons parsley, 1 1/2 teaspoons thyme, 1 1/2 teaspoons oregano, and 1 1/2 teaspoons chives.

To assemble packages, divide vegetables in to 4 portions and place them on one half of each heart. Place a piece of fish on each nest of vegetables. Sprinkle with salt, pepper, and herbs. Spoon 2 to 3 tablespoons of sundried tomato mixture (from the blender) on each portion of fish.

Begin sealing the package by folding over the other side of the heart and folding the edges inward together. Continue folding and crimping small sections until almost sealed at the pointy end. Before closing completely, ladle in 2 tablespoons each of the white wine mixture. Close and place on baking sheet. Bake for 8 to 20 minutes (depending on type and cut of fish) until done.

*Serves 4*

### *Pink Peppercorn–Crusted Seasonal Fish with Warm Gazpacho Salsa and Cucumber Water*

#### WARM GAZPACHO SALSA

2 tablespoons garlic, minced
3/4 cup diced red onion
1 cup diced celery
1 cup seeded and diced tomato
1 cup seeded and diced cucumber
1/4 cup diced red bell pepper
1/3 cup diced green bell pepper
1/4 cup diced yellow bell pepper
1 teaspoon minced jalapeño pepper
3 tablespoon chiffonnaded basil
1 teaspoon chopped oregano
1/2 teaspoon chopped thyme
1 1/2 teaspoons chopped parsley
Juice of one lemon
2 tablespoons olive oil

#### CUCUMBER WATER

2 whole cucumbers
Salt and white pepper to taste

4 (8-ounce) fillets seasonal fish (like orange roughy, cod, or trout)
3 teaspoons ground pink peppercorns
$^1/_2$ teaspoon chopped parsley
$^1/_2$ teaspoon chopped thyme
$^1/_2$ teaspoon chopped oregano
$^1/_2$ teaspoon chopped chives
Olive oil
$^1/_4$ cup white wine
$^1/_2$ cup tomato juice
Extra-virgin olive oil, for garnish

Prepare the Gazpacho Salsa: Combine garlic, red onion, celery, tomato, cucumber, bell peppers, jalapeño, basil, oregano, thyme, parsley, lemon juice and olive oil in a large bowl and toss. Set aside.

Prepare the Cucumber Water: Juice the cucumbers in a juicer or puree in a blender. Strain through a coffee filter. Season to taste with salt and white pepper and set aside.

Rub the fish with the peppercorns and the parsley, thyme, oregano, and chives, and grill. While fish is cooking, heat a sauté pan until it is very hot. Add olive oil and Gazpacho Salsa. Saute briefly; remove vegetables from the pan, add the white wine, and deglaze the pan, allowing the liquid to reduce. Add the tomato juice and allow to reduce, then remove the pan from the heat.

To serve, place the vegetable mixture in the center of a plate and place the cooked fish on top.

Pour the cucumber water around the vegetables and fish. Garnish with a drizzle of extra virgin olive oil in the cucumber water.

*Serves 4*

*Deborah Knight attended the California Culinary Academy in San Francisco. She has worked at such fine restaurants as 8700 Restaurant with Chef Cary Neff, the Miraval Health and Wellness Spa in Tucson, and the European Café in Boulder. Deborah then returned to her hometown of Scottsdale and opened her own restaurant, Mosaic. With an emphasis on culinary delights both visual and sensory, Mosaic represents the essence of the finest dining experience in Scottsdale.*

### Johnny and Mary Jo Mosca, Mosca's (New Orleans, Louisiana)

*Chicken Cacciatore*

3/4 cup olive oil
2 (3-pound) chickens, cut into eighths
1/2 teaspoon salt
1 teaspoon freshly ground black pepper
10 cloves peeled garlic, mashed
1 teaspoon rosemary
1 teaspoon oregano
1/2 cup dry white wine
1 1/2 cups tomato sauce or 1 (16-ounce) can peeled, crushed tomatoes

Heat the olive oil in a large skillet. Add the chicken pieces, turning them often, until they are browned.

Sprinkle the chicken pieces with salt and pepper. Add the garlic, rosemary, and oregano, stirring to distribute the seasonings.

Remove the pan from the stove. Pour the wine over the chicken. Add the tomato sauce or crushed, peeled tomatoes, return to the stove, and simmer 10 to 15 minutes until wine and tomatoes have blended and thickened.

*Serves 6*

*Mosca's is a very popular family-run restaurant that lies just outside New Orleans. It is owned and operated by Johnny and Mary Jo Mosca and has won the James Beard Foundation American Regional Classics Award.*

## Bernard R. Guillas, The Shores, and the La Jolla Beach and Tennis Club (San Diego, California)

### *Marine Room Maine Lobster Bisque with Enoki Mushrooms and Apricot Brandy*

2 (1¼-pound) lobsters, cooked and cooled
¼ cup olive oil
½ cup chopped celery
½ cup chopped white onion
½ cup chopped leek, white part only
2 tablespoons chopped garlic
¼ cup apricot brandy
1 cup diced tomatoes
⅓ cup tomato paste
¼ cup whole wheat flour
½ cup white wine
4 thyme sprigs
1 bay leaf
1 quart vegetable stock
¾ cup heavy cream
1 teaspoon lobster base
Sea salt to taste

Pinch cayenne pepper
1 package enoki mushrooms
1 tablespoon finely chopped chives for garnish

Remove the shells from lobster and cut the tail meat into medallions, and set the claw meat and tail medallions aside.

Coarsely chop the lobster shells and the heads. Heat the olive oil into a large, heavy kettle and brown the celery, onion, and leek over high heat. Add the lobster shells and cook 5 minutes, stirring constantly. Flambé with the brandy. Add the tomatoes, tomato paste, and flour. Cook 2 minutes, mixing well. Add wine, thyme, bay leaf, and vegetable stock and stir. Bring to boil. Reduce heat to medium and simmer fir 45 minutes.

Strain through a fine sieve, pressing on solids to attain maximum extraction and flavor. Return mixture to the pot and bring to boil. Add the heavy cream and cook 5 minutes. Season with sea salt and cayenne pepper to taste. Place soup in blender and process to smooth.

To serve, place the enoki mushrooms on base of soup plate. Pour in the lobster bisque and add the lobster-tail medallions and claw meat. Garnish with chopped chives.

*Serves 6*

*Award-winning chef Bernard R. Guillas joined the La Jolla Beach & Tennis Club as executive chef in 1994, where he directs the resort's three restaurants. Originally from Brittany, Guillas began his formal training at La Bretagne in Questembert, France, where he apprenticed with the legendary Georges Paineau. Over the next six years, he expanded his culinary knowledge with several Maitres Cuisinier de France. After coming to the United States, Guillas spent time at Maison Blanche in Washington, D.C. and the U. S. Grant Hotel in San Diego. Selected as one of fifteen rising-star chefs in 1996, he was recently awarded the 2001 Best Chef in San Diego Award from the California Restaurant Association and was inducted into the International Restaurant and Hospitality Rating Bureau's American Chefs Hall of Fame. In addition, Chef Bernard has contributed to numerous cookbooks and has made many television appearances.*

## Hans Röckenwagner, Röckenwagner Restaurant (Santa Monica, California)

### *Home-Cured Tomatoes*

I still can't believe that people buy sundried tomatoes in a supermarket. We make our own in the oven, which is inexpensive and easy. Storing them in olive oil gives them a wonderful flavor and creates an aromatic oil that is great for sautéeing and vinaigrettes. Depending on what you will be using them for, try adding a few cloves of slivered garlic to the oil. This recipe can be halved, doubled, or tripled.

1/4 cup extra-virgin olive oil
Salt and freshly ground pepper
3 pounds ripe plum tomatoes, halved (cores
    removed if woody)
2 teaspoons dried thyme or marjoram, crumbled
Extra-virgin olive oil for storing (optional)

Preheat the oven to 150°F. (This low temperature is difficult for some ovens to maintain. Be sure to use an oven thermometer and, if the oven keeps climbing up to a higher temperature, prop the oven door open about an inch with a bunched-up kitchen towel.)

Generously brush 2 baking sheets with 2 to 3 tablespoons of the olive oil and sprinkle them with salt and pepper. Arrange the halved tomatoes on the pan, cut side up, and brush them with the remaining olive oil. Sprinkle the cut sides with salt, pepper, and the herbs. Dry the tomatoes in the warm oven for 6 to 8 hours, or until they are shriveled and slightly golden, but still juicy, with a very deep and concentrated flavor. Store in an airtight container in the refrigerator for up to

1 week. If desired, cover the tomatoes with olive oil and store for up to 3 weeks.

*Yields 3 pounds tomatoes*

*Beginning his career in Germany's Black Forest, Hans Röckenwagner opened his restaurant in 1984. The* Los Angeles Times, Gourmet *magazine, the Zagat survey and the TV Food Network consistently recognize Chef Röckenwagner and his restaurant as one of the best in Southern California.*

### Roxanne Klein, Roxanne's (Larkspur, California)

#### *Crushed Blackberries with Tahitian Vanilla Bean Custard Parfait*

1 recipe Tahitian Vanilla Bean Custard (recipe below)
1 sprig lavender or fresh sweet thyme
1 pint blackberries
Date granules (to sweeten to taste)
2 tablespoons chopped dried nuts or your choice

Crush thyme or lavender in large mortar with pestle. Add blackberries and date granules to taste and gently crush together, leaving some of the berries whole.

Layer berries and cream in parfait or martini glasses and top with chopped nuts.

*Serves 4*

### Tahitian Vanilla Bean Custard

1 cup coconut meat
1 cup cashews, soaked
1/4 teaspoon tahitian vanilla bean
1/3 cup dates

Blend all ingredients together

*A graduate of the California Culinary Academy, Roxanne Klein has worked at such international-ly recognized restaurants as Stars, the Lark Creek Inn, and Le Verdon in France. Her cre-ativity with living-foods cuisine and her broad knowledge of organic ingredients has earned re-spect and rave reviews from culinary authorities and restaurant critics alike. The* San Francisco Chronicle *gave Roxanne's a rare three and a half star (out of four) rating. Roxanne is currently working with renowned chef Charlie Trotter on a living-foods cookbook.*

# Susanna Foo, Susannah Foo's
## (Philadelphia, Pennsylvania)

### *Wild Mushroom Soup*

$1/2$ ounce dried shiitake mushrooms (about 6
 medium whole)
$1/4$ pound fresh shiitake mushrooms
$1/4$ pound oyster or chanterelle mushrooms
$1/4$ pound white button mushrooms
$1/4$ cup olive oil
2 shallots, minced
1 tablespoon peeled, grated gingerroot
4 cups chicken stock
$1/2$ cup unsweetened coconut milk (I prefer the
 Chaokoh brand, which is carried by most Asian
 grocery stores)
$1/2$ teaspoon freshly ground white pepper
1 tablespoon water
1 scallion, thinly sliced, or 6 chives, chopped, plus
 more for garnish
 1 tablespoon finely chopped lemon grass (if fresh
 lemon grass is not available, substitute another
 fresh herb, such as thyme.)
1 tablespoon white vinegar or juice of 1 lemon
Coarse or kosher salt
Freshly ground pepper

Place the dried mushrooms in a bowl. Add 4 cups
lukewarm water and soak for 30 minutes, or until
softened.

Remove the mushrooms from the water; squeeze dry. Discard the water. Remove and discard the stems. Thinly slice the mushroom caps; set aside. Use a damp cloth to wipe clean all of the fresh mushrooms, keeping the button mushrooms separate. Remove the stems of the shiitake mushrooms only; discard. Cut all the mushrooms into thin slices. Heat 2 tablespoons of the oil in a large stockpot. Add the shallots and cook until lightly browned, about 2 minutes. Add the gingerroot and the dried and button mushrooms and cook, stirring, over medium heat for 3 minutes.

Add the chicken stock, coconut milk, and white pepper to the stockpot.

Add water. Mix thoroughly and stir into the soup. Bring to a boil, then reduce to a simmer. Cover and cook for 30 minutes. While the soup is cooking, heat the remaining 2 tablespoons of oil in a small skillet. Add the fresh sliced shiitake and oyster or chanterelle mushrooms and cook over high heat until soft, about 2 minutes. Keep warm until ready to use. Add the scallions or chives, lemon grass and vinegar or lemon juice to the soup. Taste to correct the seasonings. Divide the reserved mushrooms among 4 soup bowls.

Ladle the soup into the bowls and garnish with additional scallions or chives.

*Serves 4*

### Veal Chops with Mushrooms

3 tablespoons soy sauce
2 tablespoons brandy
1 tablespoon Asian sesame oil
1 tablespoon corn oil
1/2 teaspoon freshly ground pepper
4 (10- to 12-ounce) veal rib chops
5 tablespoons olive oil
2 scallions, finely chopped
3 shallots, finely chopped
1 pound mushrooms; chanterelles, shiitakes,
    oysters or white buttons, sliced thin (remove the
    stems if using shiitake or button mushrooms)
Coarse or kosher salt
Freshly ground pepper

Combine the first five ingredients in a large shallow bowl. Mix thoroughly and set aside.

Place the veal chops between 2 pieces of wax paper or plastic wrap and pound lightly to tenderize the meat. Add the meat to the marinade, turning to coat well, and refrigerate for about 20 minutes.

Preheat the broiler, with a rack 4 to 6 inches from the heat. Remove the chops from the marinade and drain well; set aside the marinade.

Heat the oil in a large skillet until very hot. Place the chops in the skillet and cook over high heat until they are lightly browned on both sides, about 2 to 3 minutes per side. Do not crowd the meat; cook the chops in 2 batches, if necessary. Do not wash the skillet.

Remove the chops from the skillet and place on the broiler rack. Broil for 3 to 5 minutes, turning once, for medium-rare meat. You can cook the chops for 1 to 2 minutes more if you prefer your meat well done. Meanwhile, reheat the skillet. Add the scallions and the shallots and cook over high heat, strring, until they are lightly browned, 2 to 3 minutes.

Add the mushrooms and mix well to coat with the oil. Add the reserved veal marinade and cook, stirring for 2 to 3 minutes, or until the mushrooms are just cooked. Season to taste with salt and pepper. When the chops are done, divide them among 4 serving plates and top with the mushrooms and the sauce.

*Serves 4*

*Susanna Foo's unique cuisine has won praise from critics and food lovers around the country. In 1995, Susanna's first cookbook,* Susanna Foo Chinese Cuisine, *received rave reviews from magazines, newspapers, and radio. In 1996, the book won the James Beard Foundation award for Best International Cookbook. In 1997, Susanna became the first chef in Pennsylvania to win the most prestigious James Beard Foundation award for Best Chef in the Mid-Atlantic Region. Additionally, in 1998, Susanna Foo Chinese Cuisine was recognized by the Philadelphia Inquirer with the first four-bell rating in Philadelphia. The restaurant was among the top five most popular restaurants in Philadelphia in the Zagat Survey from 1998 through 2002. The restaurant was awarded the AAA four-diamond award from 1999 through 2002 and the Mobil four-star award from 1998 through 2002.*

### Gilbert Garza, Suze Restaurant
### (Dallas, Texas)

#### *Artichoke Pesto*

2 (10-ounce) jars of brined artichoke hearts
1¹/₂ cups of grated pecorino romano cheese
¹/₄ cup of garlic puree
Juice of 4 to 5 lemons
1 cup of extra virgin olive oil
Salt to taste
2 tablespoons of cracked black pepper

Start by squeezing out all of the excess liquid from the artichokesand set aside. Juice the lemons and add half to the artichokes, then fold and mix in the romano, the garlic, and the olive oil. Season with salt and the cracked black pepper, and the other half of the lemon juice. Serve chilled as a salad or as a cold appetizer.

*Serves 6 to 8*

*Twenty-four years ago, Gilbert Garza began working in his grandfather's restaurant. After graduating from the California Culinary Academy, Garza worked alongside Chef Kent Rathbun at the Landmark restaurant and at The Mansion on Turtle Creek with Dean Fearing. He opened his own restaurant, Toscana, in 1996. Toscana was named a* D Magazine *Best New Restaurant winner and One of the Top Italian Restaurants in North America by* USA Today. D Magazine *ranked his new restaurant, Suze, among the Top Ten New Restaurants for 1999. Suze was also named a Top Ten New Restaurant by Jim White of the KRLD Radio Food Show.*

## Gary Coyle, Tavern on the Green
### (New York City)

### *Marinated Goat Cheese with Grilled Asparagus Salad with Bicolored Tomato Vinaigrette*

MARINATED GOAT CHEESE

8-ounce log goat cheese
4 tablespoons chopped fresh herbs, such as cilantro, rosemary, and parsley
3 tablespoons Crisco Vegetable Oil
1 tablespoon olive oil
Balsamic vinegar
Kosher salt and pepper to taste

GRILLED ASPARAGUS SALAD

1 bunch medium asparagus (approximately 20 to 24 pieces)
Crisco No-Stick Cooking Spray
Kosher salt and pepper to taste

BICOLORED TOMATO VINAIGRETTE

1 large ripe red tomato
1 large ripe yellow tomato
$1/8$ cup red wine vinegar or cider vinegar
$1/4$ cup Crisco Vegetable Oil
$1/4$ cup virgin olive oil
Kosher salt and pepper

Prepare the Marinated Goat Cheese: Roll the goat cheese in the chopped herbs. Place in a flat glass pan with the Crisco Vegetable Oil, olive oil, vinegar, salt, and pepper. Coat the cheese; cover and set aside at room temperature for 15 minutes.

Prepare the Grilled Asparagus: Preheat the broiler. Make a single layer of asparagus on a flame-proof pan. Spray with Crisco No-Stick Cooking Spray and season with salt and pepper. Place under the broiler and cook for several minutes until the asparagus slightly chars. Remove and set aside at room temperature.

Prepare the Tomato Vinaigrette: Cut the tomatoes in half and squeeze out the seeds. Cut each half into 1/4-inch dice. Combine with vinegar, Crisco Vegetable Oil, and olive oil. Season with salt and pepper.

To assemble the salad, fan 4 or 5 pieces of asparagus on each plate. Cut the goat cheese into 4 pieces and place one piece at the bottom of the stems of asparagus. Drizzle the remaining marinade over the cheese. Spoon the Tomato Vinaigrette over the asparagus. Serve immediately.

*Serves 4*

## *Panache of Shrimp and Scallops with Cucumber Vermicelli and Lobster-Bacon Casino Butter*

### LOBSTER-BACON CASINO BUTTER

4 slices bacon (about 4 ounces)

1/4 cup softened butter

4 tablespoons diced shallots

2 cloves garlic, minced

1/4 cup finely diced green peppers

1/4 cup heavy cream

2 tablespoons rough-chopped flat parsley

1/4 cup diced cooked lobster meat

Juice of 2 lemons (about 3 tablespoons)

1/4 teaspoon kosher salt

Freshly ground black pepper

### FOR THE SHELLFISH

16 jumbo shrimp, peeled, deveined, tail on, and
   butterflied

16 large sea scallops (connecting tissue removed).

16 large toothpicks (to skewer the shrimp)

3 tablespoons olive oil

2 tablespoons softened butter

1 large seedless cucumber, peeled and thinly sliced
   spaghetti-style

3 tablespoons olive oil

1 cup sauteed, seasoned spinach (warm)

Preheat the oven to 375°F.

In a medium skillet over medium heat, cook the bacon to a crisp. Reserving the drippings, allow the bacon to cool and roughly chop it. Melt the butter and add the bacon drippings. Sweat the shallots, garlic and green pepper; add the cream, and reduce by 1/3 until thick. Stir in the parsley, lobster, lemon juice and season with salt and pepper. Remove from the pan and keep warm.

Skewer the shrimp and scallops with the toothpicks. Brush with olive oil and season with salt and pepper. Place on a baking pan and roast 10 to 12 minutes until the scallops are cooked. Remove from oven and transfer the shrimp and scallops to a platter and keep warm.

In a saute pan, melt the butter and saute the cucumber. Gently season with salt and pepper.

In the center of each of four plates, evenly divde the spinach. Top each with 1/4 of the cucumber mixture. Remove the toothpicks from the shrimp and scallops and place 4 shrimp and scallops at 4 points around the spinach-cucumber mixture. Drizzle the sauce over and serve immediately.

*Serves 4*

## Tavern Crabcakes with Avocado Tartar Sauce

2 pounds lump crabmeat
1/4 cup mayonnaise
3 tablespoons white wine
1/4 cup chopped scallion
3 tablespoons Old Bay seasoning
4 eggs, beaten,
1 tablespoon Worcestershire sauce
1 teaspoon hot sauce
1 cup whole-wheat flour
2 eggs, beaten
2 cups whole grain breadcrumbs
3 cups baby or regular washed and dried arugula
Juice of 1 lemon
2 tablespoons olive oil
Salt and pepper to taste
1 recipe Avocado Tartar Sauce (recipe below)

Gently mix the crabmeat, mayonnaise, scallions, Old Bay, 4 eggs, Worcestershire sauce, and hot sauce. Form into 8 cakes. Dredge each cake in the whole-wheat flour, dip in the 2 beaten eggs, and then dredge in the whole-grain breadcrumbs. Deep-fry or sauté cakes until done. Keep warm.

In a large bowl, toss together the arugula, lemon juice, and salt and pepper.

To serve, place two crabcakes on each plate, dress with the arugula salad, and top with the Avocado Tartar Sauce.

*Serves 4*

AVOCADO TARTAR SAUCE

1 ripe avocado, mashed
1 hard boiled egg, chopped
1/4 cup mayonnaise
1 tablespoon chopped sweet pickle
3 tablespoon sour cream
1 tablespoon each chopped parsley, chervil, chives
1 tablespoon lemon juice
1 tablespoon capers
1/8 teaspoon cayenne

Combind the above ingredients in a small bowl.

*Gary Coyle has held top positions at such fine dining establishments as the St. Francis Hotel in San Francisco, the Meridien Hotel, La Cote Basque, and the Rainbow Room in New York City and Rittenhouse Hotel in Philadelphia. He is currently the executive chef at the renowned Tavern on the Green in New York City.*

**Tony Vallone, Vallone Restaurant Group
(Tony's, Anthony's, La Griglia, Grotto,
Los Tonyos, Houston, Texas)**

### Layered Asian Tuna

4 (7-ounce) portions cooked yellowfin tuna
4 whole roasted tomatoes, sliced in half
8 tablespoons Soy Onions (recipe below)
4 pinches daikon sprouts
2 teaspoons finely julienned pickled beets
Pinch toasted white and black sesame seeds
4 teaspoons wasabi
8 teaspoons sliced green onions
Ponzu Vinaigrette (recipe below)

Sear the tuna so it is rare, and cut each portion
horizontally into three equal pieces. On each
plate, place a layer of tuna, top that with roasted
tomatoes, add a second layer of tuna, top that with
a layer of Soy Onions, and top with the last piece
of tuna. Do this for each of the four servings.

Garnish each serving with a pinch of daikon
sprouts, a half-teaspoon of pickled beets, a pinch
of sesame seeds, a teaspoon of wasabi, sliced green
onions, and a splash of Ponzu Vinaigrette.

*Serves 4*

SOY ONIONS

3 to 4 medium red onions, sliced thin
1 cup sake
1 cup rice wine vinegar
1 cup light soy sauce
1 tablespoon minced garlic
1 tablespoon chopped fresh ginger

Combine all ingredients together and reduce in a saucepan over medium flame until almost dry. Store covered in the refrigerator.

PONZU VINAIGRETTE

3/4 cup light soy sauce
1/8 cup sesame oil
3/4 cup rice wine vinegar
2 limes, juice
2 cups vegetable oil
Salt and pepper

Combine all ingredients together and mix well.

## Whole-Wheat Linguine with Crab and Shrimp

3 tablespoon extra virgin olive oil
1 tablespoon slivered garlic
8 ounces small fresh shrimp, cleaned and peeled
1 cup crushed Italian tomatoes
1 tablespoon chopped Italian parsley
Salt, pepper, and crushed red pepper to taste
2 cups chopped fresh tomato
1/3 cup julienned fresh basil
1 pound jumbo lump crabmeat
1 pound whole-wheat linguine, cooked

In a large sauté pan, add olive oil and garlic cook about 45 seconds on medium heat. Add the shrimp and cook 3 to 4 minutes; add the crushed tomatoes and cook about 4 to 5 minutes longer. Add the parsley and season with salt and pepper. Add 1/2 of the basil and the crabmeat. Heat crab through for about 3 minutes (be very careful not to stir too much so you won't break the crab). Take a little sauce and mix with cooked linguine and toss.

Put into alarge bowl and top with sauce and garnish with remaining basil.

*Serves 6*

As Houston institutions, the restaurants that make up the Vallone Restaurant Group are as diverse as they are delicious, attracting locals as well as visiting celebrities and Houston society. They all share a commitment to outstanding cuisine based on the finest ingredients and most innovative recipes. All of the restaurants have won numerous national awards. Tony Vallone is supporter of many civic and national philanthropic causes, as well as the author of *Tony's: The Cookbook.* Tony is also an ardent follower of the Sugar Busters! *lifestyle, and his menus feature whole wheat breads, flatbreads, crepes, pastas, and tortillas.*

# Patricia Radicevic, Three Brothers Restaurant (Milwaukee, Wisconsin)

## *Peppers Stuffed with Rice and Veggies*

3 or 4 tablespoon extra-virgin olive oil, plus more
  for pan
3/4 cup finely diced onion
3 cups chicken stock or water
2 cups brown rice, rinsed and drained
1 teaspoon salt
12 to 14 medium-size green bell peppers
1 zucchini, peeled and coarsely grated
1 carrot, peeled and coarsely grated
2 teaspoon dried dill
3 or 4 teaspoons (or to taste) finely minced garlic
Salt and black pepper to taste
2 or 3 tomatoes (cut in sixths), optional
1 cup water

Preheat the oven to 375°F.

In a stockpot over low to moderate heat, saute the onions in the oil until they are transparent. Add the chicken stock or water and bring to a boil. Add the rice and salt, and return to a boil. Reduce heat, cover tightly, and simmer over low heat until the rice is tender (approximately 20 to 25 minutes).

Empty the rice into a mixing bowl and allow it to cool. Cut a thin slice from the stem end of each pepper (saving the tops to act as lids, if desired), remove the seeds and membranes, wash, and drain upside down.

When rice is cool, add zucchini, carrot, dill, garlic, and salt and pepper to taste, and mix well. Add olive oil to mixture to moisten and further bind the rice. Fill the peppers with rice and cover tops either with pepper lids or tomato chunks.

Grease with a little olive oil the bottom of a roasting pan large enough to hold peppers upright. Add 1 cup of water to the pan. Place peppers upright in the pan and cover tightly with foil. Bake for about 1 1/2 hours or until tender.

*Yields 12 to 14 peppers*

*Patricia Radicevic has spent thirty years in the restaurant business and her schooling consists solely of on-the-job training. With her husband, Branko, she carefully prepares and preserves the Serbian recipes passed down by her mother-in-law. In 2002, they received the James Beard Foundation's America's Regional Classics Award. They have also been recognized in such publications as* Gourmet, Bon Appetit, *and* The New York Times.

Rosewood Hotels and Resorts owns and manages some of the most exquisite establishments around the world. These include The Carlyle Hotel in New York City, The Mansion on Turtle Creek in Dallas, Al Faisaliah Hotel in Riyadh, Saudi Arabia, Caneel Bay in St. John, U.S. Virgin Islands, The Dharmawansanga in Jakarta, Indonesia, Hotel Crescent Court in Dallas, Hotel Seiyo Ginza in Tokyo, Japan, Las Ventanas al Paraiso in Los Cabos, Mexico, and Little Dix Bay in Virgin Gorda, the British Virgin Islands.

Below are the best recipes from the fine restaurants at these outstanding hotels and resorts.

## Warren Pearson, Al Faisaliah
## (Riyadh, Saudi Arabia)

### *Fillet of Beef Marinated with Japanese Spices*

8 ounces beef tenderloin

Juice of 1 lemon

6 ounces leeks, white part only, cut into 1³/₄-inch
   lengths

3 ounces oyster mushrooms

4 ounces curly endive and oak leaf lettuce, washed
   and dried well

Salt and freshly ground pepper

Roasted sesame seeds

Shoga (pickled sliced ginger)

DRESSING

1 tablespoon Wasabi (or to taste)
2 tablespoons sherry vinegar
2 tablespoon white wine vinegar
6 tablespoon Kikkoman soy sauce
Freshly ground black pepper
1 teaspoon grated ginger
1 teaspoon chives chopped
1 tablespoon honey

Cut the beef fillet into thin slices and, layered between sheets of plastic film, carefully beat until extremely thin. Sprinkle the meat with about half the lemon juice, and some salt and pepper.

Cook the leek with remaining lemon juice and some salt in boiling water until just tender, then drain.

Mix together the dressing ingredients, then marinate the leeks while still warm with 1/3 dressing.

Season the oyster mushrooms with salt and pepper and sauté them quickly until brown in a nonstick pan.

Arrange the dry salad leaves and the leek on individual serving plates, and carefully arrange the thin meat slices on top.

Garnish with the still warm oyster mushrooms.

Top with rest of dressing and garnish with roasted sesame and pickled ginger.

*Serves 4*

## Ray Henry, Caneel Bay
### (St. John, U.S. Virgin Islands)

### *Chili-Roasted Calamari*

Olive oil
2 pounds sliced squid bodies
2 cloves of garlic, minced
1/2 teaspoon chili flakes
8 seeded plum tomatoes, peeled and diced
1/4 cup toasted pine nuts
1/4 cup julienned black olives
2 tablespoons pesto
Juice of 1 lemon
1/4 cup butter
2 tablespoons balsamic vinegar
Fresh basil julienne for garnish

In a skillet, heat oil until smoking. Add squid and sauté for 1 to 2 minutes. Remove squid from pan and keep warm.

Add the garlic and chili flakes and cook until golden. Add the tomatoes and cook until quite dry. Toss in the pine nuts and black olives. Add the squid and cook for 2 minutes. Add the pesto and season to taste. Add the lemon juice and the butter, season with the vinegar, and serve in small bowls with basil julienne as garnish.

*Serves 8*

## Jean Louis Dumonet, The Carlyle
## (New York City)

### Cassoulet

2 cups Great Northern dried beans
2 duck legs confit (with some fat), halved*
1/4 pound slab bacon, diced
3 to 4 garlic cloves, minced
1 bouquet garni**
4 to 6 cups chicken stock
2 to 3 ounces smoked ham, cut into large pieces
1/4 pound garlic sausage, cut into 4 slices*
2 cups fresh whole-grain bread crumbs

Soak the beans in cold water overnight. Drain well.

Preheat oven to 425°F. Place a tablespoon or so of the fat surrounding the duck legs in a large, ovenproof pot with a lid. Add the bacon and cook on the stove top, over medium heat, stirring often, until softened, 3 to 5 minutes. Stir in the garlic and cook until softened but not browned, 1 to 2 minutes longer. Add the beans and the bouquet garni.

Pour 4 cups of the stock, season to taste with salt, increase heat to high and bring to a boil. Cover and transfer to the oven.

Cook, covered, until the beans are tender, about

1¹/₂ hours. Stir often to prevent sticking. Add additional stock if necessary to prevent drying out.

Place the ham, sliced sausage, and confit in the bottom of a 1¹/₂- to 2-quart ovenproof serving dish. Fill with the beans. Top with the bread crumbs and return to the oven. Cook for 20 minutes or until golden brown on top and heated through.

Serve at once.

* Duck confit and garlic sausage are available from D' Artagnan, Inc. at 1-800-DARTAGNAN.
** For a bouquet garni: Tie 3 parsley sprigs, 2 sprigs of fresh thyme and a bay leaf together with kitchen string in a piece of cheesecloth.

*Serves 4*


### Jean-Marie Dubos, Hotel Crescent (Dallas, Texas)


### *Grilled Salmon with Vegetable Terrine and Kalamata Olive Vinaigrette*

4 (5-ounce) salmon steaks
Pea tendrils (for garnish)
Lemon oil (for garnish)
Dried olives (for garnish)

MARINADE

2 tablespoons paprika
4 tablespoons mustard seeds
1 tablespoons cumin seeds
1 tablespoons garlic powder
1 tablespoons coriander seeds
6 ounces olive oil

VEGETABLE TERRINE

Olive oil
Balsamic vinegar
1 teaspoon chopped fresh oregano
2 teaspoons chopped fresh thyme, divided
salt and pepper to taste
12 slices zucchini, straight cut
12 slices Japanese eggplant, straight cut
12 slices yellow squash, straight cut
32 pieces julienned roasted red pepper
2 ounces goat cheese
2 ounces mascarpone cheese

KALAMATA OLIVE VINAIGRETTE

3 cups balsamic vinegar
1 bunch of blanched basil leaves
1 ounce chopped shallots
1/2 ounce garlic, peeled and roughly chopped
1 cup kalamata olives
4 ounces olive juice
Salt and pepper to taste
1 1/2 cups olive oil

Prepare the marinade: Toast the paprika, mustard seeds, cumin seeds, garlic poweder, and coriander seeds in a sauté pan. Do not burn; lightly heat until the spices give off an aromatic perfume. Blend in the olive oil.

Add the salmon to the marinade and refrigerate for at least 12 hours.

Prepare the Vegetable Terrine: Combine the olive oil and balsamic vinegar, oregano, 1 teaspoon thyme, and salt and pepper. Marinate all the vegetables this mixture for 45 minutes. Meanwhile, mix together the goat cheese, the mascarpone cheese, and the remaining teaspoon of thyme. Grill the vegetables on both sides until fully cooked. Stack 4 pieces of each vegetables in a 3-inch ring mold starting with the yellow squash, then the roasted red bell pepper, then the cheese mixture, then the eggplant, and then the zucchini. Lightly press the stack to compress.

Prepare the Vinaigrette: In a blender, process the vinegar, basil, shallots, garlic, olives, olive juice, and salt and pepper. Slowly add the olive oil to emulsify, and refrigerate until ready to use.

Grill the marinated salmon until done. To serve, place one slice of vegetable terrine on each plate and heat it in the microwave for 15 seconds. Remove and add the salmon; drizzle the vinaigrette around the plate. Garnish with pea tendrils, lemon oil, and dried olives.

## Chris Janssens, The Dharmawangsa
### (Jakarta, Indonesia)

### *Roast Fennel and Olive Salad*

4 baby fennel bulbs, quartered
2 red onions, each cut into eight pieces
4 plum tomatoes, halved
3 tablespoons olive oil
2 tablespoons oregano leaves
Beet leaves or salad greens
1 cup Ligurian olives (or other small olives)

Dressing

3 tablespoon apple cider vinegar
2 teaspoon Dijon mustard
2 tablespoon olive oil
1 clove garlic, crushed

Preheat the oven to 400°F.

Place the fennel, onions, and tomatoes in a baking dish. Heat the oil in a small saucepan over low heat. Add oregano to pan and cook for 3 minutes. Pour the oil and oregano over the vegetables and bake for 30 minutes.

To make the dressing, whisk together the vinegar, mustard, oil and garlic.

To serve, place vegetables on a bed of baby beet or salad greens on serving plates. Sprinkle salad with olives and dressing.

# Shoji Hirota, Hotel Seiyo Ginza (Tokyo, Japan)

## *Warm Tart of Ripe Tomato with Eggplant Caviar and Basil*

4 ripe tomatoes
4 pack phyllo dough
Olive oil

SET A

1/2 onion, sliced
1/2 garlic clove
1 sprig thyme
1 bay leaf
1 tablespoon olive oil
salt and pepper to taste

SET B

2 slices semidried tomato, chopped
1/4 teaspoons herbes de provence
2 leaves basil, chopped
1/5 garlic clove
4 black olives, chopped

SET C

4 pounds of eggplant
1 1/4 cups olive oil (for roasting)
2 tablespoons extra-virgin olive
1 1/2 tablespoons anchovy fillets

5¹/₂ tablespoons black olive paste
1 tablespoon chopped garlic
salt and pepper to taste

SET D

5 basil leaves
3 tablespoons olive oil

Preheat the oven to 350°F.

Cut the phyllo sheets into 4-inch rounds. Brush olive oil onto the phyllo and make 5 to 6 layers. Place on a baking tray, add some weight on it, and bake for 7 to 8 minutes.

Put all ingredients in Set A in a cocotte, wrap it, and cook it until all ingredients are nicely soft. Remove the thyme, bay leaf, and garlic.

Add the ingredients from Set B to those of Set A and mix them.

Set C: Cut the eggplant lengthwise in half, cut the white meat of the eggplant without cutting the skin, add olive oil and salt, and bake it until it goes soft. Chill the eggplant and mash it to create a paste. Add other ingredients.

Set D: Put ingredients in a mixer and make a pistou.

Spread a mix of B and A onto the phyllo dough and add some ¹/₄-inch-thick thick slices of tomato. Bake it for 8 minutes. When serving, add the eggplant paste onto the dish and some fresh basil leaves on top.

The pistou can be sprinkled around the dish for additional flavor and beauty.


## *Pan-Fried Prawns with Green Vegetables*

8 (6-ounce) prawns
Salt and white pepper
1 cup cream
1 cup flour
2 tablespoons butter
2 ounces green beans, boiled until crisp-tender
2 ounces snow peas, boiled until crisp-tender
1 tablespoon chopped shallots
2 tablespoons hazelnut oil
$1/3$ cup unsweetened whipped cream
2 tablespoons yogurt
1 tablespoon chives
2 teaspoons chopped shallots
Lemon juice to taste


Slightly spice the prawns with salt and white pepper to taste. Dip the prawns into the cream, dredge with flour, and fry in butter.

Cut the green beans and snow peas $1/2$-inch-long pieces. Put in a bowl; add chopped shallots, hazelnut oil, salt and pepper to taste, and mix.

Combine whipped cream, yogurt, salt, pepper, lemon juice, chopped chives, and shallots.

Put the warm vegetables each plate, place 2 prawns in the center of each plate, and spoon the cream around each.

*Serves 4*

## Marc Lippman, Las Ventanas al Paraiso (Los Cabos, Mexico)

### *Mango and Jicama Salad*

16 ($^1$/3-inch thick) mango slices
16 ($^1$/3-inch thick) jicama slices
1 cup assorted fresh herbs (italian parsley, tarragon, cilantro, chives, flowering herbs)
2 tablespoons extra-virgin olive oil
Salt and pepper to taste
Habanero Vinaigrette (recipe below)

Cut the mango and jicama into 4-inch by 4-inch squares. On each plate, starting with the jicama and alternating with the mango, build a tower containing 4 slices of each.

Lightly toss the assorted fresh herbs with the olive oil and season with salt and pepper. Garnish each tower with the herbs and drizzle with the Habanero Vinaigrette.

*Serves 4*

HABANERO VINAIGRETTE

1 habanero pepper, finely diced and seeds removed
6 tablespoons extra-virgin olive oil
2 tablespoons lime juice
16 lime sections
Salt and pepper to taste

Combine all ingredients in a mixing bowl and mix well.

### Michael Rauter, Little Dix Bay
### (British Virgin Islands)

*Little Dix Bay's Seared Caribbean Swordfish Steak, with Curried Lentils, Eggplant Caviar, and Red Pepper Coulis*

SWORDFISH

1 tablespoon caribbean jerk seasoning
2 tablespoons vegetable oil
1/4 teaspoon finely chopped garlic
4 (6-ounce) swordfish steaks
salt and fresh ground black pepper to taste

CURRIED LENTILS

1/2 cup red lentils, rinsed and drained
2 slices apple-wood-smoked bacon, cut in half
1/4 onion, diced

$^1/_2$ cup diced celery root
1 cup chicken or vegetable stock
$^1/_4$ cup heavy cream
1 tablespoon madras curry powder
2 tablespoons butter
salt and freshly milled black pepper to taste

### EGGPLANT CAVIAR

1 roasted eggplant, peeped and chopped
2 tablsepoons olive oil
2 tablespoons finely chopped red onion
2 tablespoons of finely chopped peeled tomatoes
4 tablespoons cucumber, peeled, seeded & fine
  diced
1 tablespoon chopped parsley
$1^1/_2$ teaspoons chopped mint
1 garlic clove, finely chopped
Juice of one lemon
Salt and fresh ground black pepper to taste

### RED BELL PEPPER COULIS

1 red bell pepper, seeded and diced
1 tablespoon chopped ginger
2 tablespoons diced onion
2 large tomatos, peeled, quarterd, and flesh
  removed
1 tablespoon vegetable oil
$^3/_4$ cup vegetable or chicken stock
Salt and black pepper to taste

Sprig fresh mint, for garnish
Fresh chives, for garnish

Preheat the oven to 350°F.

Prepare the swordfish: Mix the jerk seasoning, the vegetable oil, and the garlic and rub the fish on all sides with the mixture. Season with salt and pepper and sauté the steaks on both sides. Transfer fish to a pan and finish in the oven, cooking for 5 to 6 minutes or until done. Set aside and keep warm.

Prepare the Curried Lentils: Melt the butter in a pan and sauté the onions with the bacon until translucent. Add the curry powder and sauté for another two minutes to release the flavor, taking care not to burn the curry. Add the celeriac and lentils, then deglaze with the chicken or vegetable stock. Simmer on low heat until lentils are done. Add the heavy cream and season with salt and pepper. Remove the Bacon and transfer the lentils to a food processor. Pulse the mixture roughly for two to five seconds, until pureed just a little, but still chunky and firm in consistency. Set aside and keep warm.

Prepare the Eggplant Caviar: In a large bowl, mix all ingredients. Chill and set aside.

Prepare the Red Bell Pepper Coulis: Heat the oil in a saucepan, add the onions, and sauté until translucent. Add the ginger, pepper, tomatoes and continue sautéing for two minutes. Deglaze with the chicken or vegetable stock and simmer until peppers are soft.

Season to taste and and pour into a blender and process until smooth. Pour through a fine sieve, adjust seasoning, set aside, and keep warm.

To serve, place some curried lentils in the center of each plate, place a piece of swordfish on top of it, and top with eggplant caviar. Drizzle the coulis around the fish and garnish with fresh mint and chives and freshly ground black pepper.

*Serves 4*

### Little Dix Bay's Roasted Pepper Salad With Tuna Fish Confit and Hummus

#### TUNA FISH CONFIT

1 pound yellowfin tuna
3 teaspoons coarse sea salt
3/4 cup vegetable oil
3/4 cup olive oil
2 garlic cloves
1/2 bay leaf
4 tablespoons crushed ginger
2 pieces star anise
1/2 cinnamon stick
1 sprig of rosemary
1 sprig of thyme
1 1/2 teaspoons black peppercorns

MARINADE

2 tablespoons olive oil
Splash of lemon juice
Splash of sesame oil
2 dried apricots, finely diced
Splash of balsamic vinegar
salt and pepper to taste


HUMMUS

1 cup chickpeas, washed and soaked overnight in
   water
3 cups chickpea soaking water
1/3 cup tahini
1/2 cup olive oil
1/2 cup lemon juice
2 cloves garlic, crushed
Salt to taste


ROASTED BELL PEPPER SALAD

1 grilled yellow pepper, cooled, skin removed, and
   julienned
1 grilled red bell pepper, cooled, skin removed, and
   julienned
1/4 pcs. red onion, fine diced
2 tablespoons balsamic vinegar
2 tablespoons olive oil
2 tablespoons roasted pine nuts

1 pinch julienned basil leaves
Salt and fresh ground black pepper to taste

FOR THE GARNISH

Fresh mint sprigs
Lavosh bread
Cooked chickpeas
Olive oil
Fresh ground black pepper

Prepare the Tuna: Sprinkle fish with sea salt and allow to rest, chilled, for 4 hours.

Heat the vegetable and olive oils on a high flame. Carefully place the fish and the rest of the ingredients in the oil and and immediately turn off the heat under the pan. Let the fish slow-cook in the hot oil and allow it to cool down to room temperature. Meanwhile, prepare the marinade by combining all the ingredients in a large bowl. Remove the fish from the oil, pat it dry, break it into rough chunks and marinate. Set aside in the refrigerator.

Prepare the Hummus: Boil the chickpeas gently in 3 cups of soaking water until tender. Place them in a food processor or blender, add the rest of the ingredients, and process until smooth. Set aside to chill.

Prepare the Roasted Bell Pepper Salad: Combine the peppers and the rest of the ingredients and set aside to chill.

To serve, place a 3-inch ring mold in the center of each plate and fill it halfway with the marinated tuna salad. Top with the bell pepper salad and remove the mold. Using two tablespoons, place a dollop of the hummus on top of the unmolded tuna and pepper salad. Garnish with mint, Lavosh bread, and chickpeas; drizzle olive oil over the salad and the plate. Finish with black pepper to taste.

*Serves 4*

### Dean Fearing, The Mansion on Turtle Creek (Dallas, Texas)

*Texas Black Bean Soup*

1 cup dry black beans
1 onion, chopped
3 cloves garlic, chopped
1 jalapeno chili, seeded and chopped
1 small leek (white part only), chopped
1 stalk celery, chopped
4 sprigs fresh cilantro
1 quart chicken stock
1 cup ham scraps or 1 large ham bone
Salt to taste
Ground black pepper to taste
Juice of 1 lemon

Rinse beans and discard any that are shriveled. Cook beans in cold water to cover for 2 to 3 hours; drain.

Place soaked beans, onion, garlic, chili, leek, celery, cilantro, chicken stock, and ham, in a large stock pot and bring to a boil over high heat. Lower heat and simmer for about 2 hours or until beans are very soft, skimming off foam frequently.

When beans are soft, remove ham scraps or bone. Pour beans into a blender or food processor (divide in batches if necessary) and blend until smooth. Strain and season to taste with salt, pepper, and lemon juice. Soup should be thick, but if it is too thick, thin with additional hot chicken stock.

# 29 | Myths

One thing we would like to do is dispel some of the concepts that have been around for so long that they are almost universally believed, even by the majority of doctors. The truth is that most doctors, dietitians, and other health professionals know very little about the complicated interplay of carbohydrates, fats, and proteins once these foods enter the body. This is an area where dogma has held sway or views have been conveniently retained, for many years and only a few individuals have challenged these misconceptions. Let's examine some of these views more closely.

## Calories and Weight Loss

What exactly is a calorie, and is it so important? A calorie is the amount of energy (heat) needed to raise the temperature of 1 kilogram of water 1 degree centigrade (from 15°C to 16°C). In other words, it is a measure of the amount of energy required to achieve a certain result. But how does this relate to the human body, and what does it mean for us?

If we were all internal combustion engines or boilers, then it would be easy to see how this concept would be important, because whatever amount of fuel went into our engine would come out as approximately an equivalent amount of energy. Theoretically, if one consumed an amount of food containing a certain number of calories, the body would have to expend this energy in a given period of time to remain calorie-neutral. If not, the assumption has always been that the body will convert these excess calories into stored energy (fat) that would be released at a later date, when the body would need more energy than it had consumed. This has been the standard theory for decades, and unfortunately, has been well accepted by most nutritional professionals. In this model, as calorie requirements are exceeded by intake, fat will undoubtedly accumulate.

Most of these premises were based on research performed decades ago, research that was not verified by other investigators or subjected to the type of scrutiny and continued refinement that are usual with most scientific research performed today. Webb reviewed a number of studies and determined that energy intake (calories) is not sufficient to predict weight gain or loss in any given individual.[1] Nevertheless, the caloric theory is widely accepted and has become deeply ingrained in the public psyche.

Fortunately, individuals have not evolved like engines, and caloric requirements and consumption never were meant to be in perfect equilibrium or so finely balanced that we should be overly concerned about small variations in either direction. In human beings, body weight is regulated by integrated and well-coordinated mechanisms that seek a dynamic balance between food intake and energy expenditure, and the truth is that no one quite yet understands exactly how the body achieves this complex process. We now know that decreasing the amount of calories in the diet only leads to temporary weight loss, so there has to be a compensating process or another explanation.

Research has shown that when we diet and lose weight, the body adjusts its energy requirements downward and thus needs to expend less energy to run itself.[2] This presents a form of resistance to maintaining a reduced weight even while maintaining exactly the same low-calorie diet. This startling phenomenon accounts for the poor long-term results of most dietary treatments of obesity. We also get miserable eating less, and few of us will voluntarily live with deprivation for the remainder of our lives—we will ultimately give in to one of life's greatest pleasures, which is eating in normal quantities.

Our view is that calories per se are not as important as the type of foods we eat, how we eat them, and what metabolic processes control their assimilation. What we do know is that normal, even significant, amounts of the proper types of food can be consumed for indefinite periods without causing weight gain!

## Fats and Weight Gain

Because fats provide more calories per gram (9) than either carbohydrates or protein (4), it has always been a popular myth that fats are bad. This has been driven in large part by the calorie-counting myth, that is, fat grams result in more calories than carbohydrate grams; therefore, eating fewer fat and more carbohydrate grams will result in consuming fewer overall calories and a healthier diet. This reasoning has given tremendous impetus to the consumption of certain types of carbohydrates, such as pasta, potatoes, and rice. This trend has now reached unprecedented proportions in this country with the current pasta craze.

The fact is that fats, in and of themselves, do not necessarily cause weight gain. Moreover, fats are vitally important to the body in many ways, from the production of hormones to the absorption of vitamins. It is true that many of us consume more fat than we need, but this is largely due to the fact that fats are present in so many food items that have become popular in this country, such as doughnuts, fried chicken, and french fries. Therefore, although consumption of a reasonable amount of fat is healthy, we agree that it is generally necessary to trim the large amount of saturated fats consumed in the normal American diet.

As the ingestion of fats as well as carbohydrates may lead to changes in cholesterol, it is very important to point out that some fats lower cholesterol and others raise it. For instance, mono-unsaturated fatty acids (contained in foods such as olive oil, canola oil, peanut oil, and pecans) may in fact be helpful for patients with coronary artery disease or with a high risk of developing coronary disease.

Reliable studies have confirmed that low rates of coronary artery disease occur in Mediterranean countries, where the population consumes a large percentage of their calories as these monounsaturated fats, primarily in the form of olive oil. Other studies show similar beneficial effects for walnuts and almonds, both rich in monounsaturated fats.[3]

However, saturated fats and many polyunsaturated fats are believed to lead to an increased risk for development of coronary disease. In a recent study where patients were randomly assigned to receive a Mediterranean-type diet that was high in vegetables, fresh fruit, whole grains, and olive oil, compared to a standard diet, there was a 79 percent decrease in major cardiovascular events after twenty-seven months in the Mediterranean group.[4] Yet the standard diet recommended for patients with or at risk for coronary disease is to consume 70 percent to

85 percent of calories from carbohydrates, with very low amounts of fat and protein! It is very possible that this may be the wrong recommendation for many patients, because such a diet can actually increase triglyceride levels and decrease high-density lipoprotein (HDL) cholesterol, the "protective" cholesterol (the higher the HDL, the better).

Another class of fats that may be beneficial for heart disease is the omega-3 polyunsaturated fatty acids, found in fish oils and flaxseed. These oils decrease triglyceride levels and decrease the stickiness of platelets in the bloodstream. Elevated triglycerides and "sticky" platelets can contribute to arteriosclerosis.

Our view, then, is that not all fats are the same, and they should not be considered as having the same effect when eaten. Many, in fact, are actually good for you, and are covered in Chapter 26.

## Cholesterol

A closely related myth is the cholesterol story. Cholesterol was not a major consideration until the early 1970s. At that time guidelines were first issued in the United States warning against the dangers of butter, eggs, lard, and other animal fats. This produced the current trend of classifying foods as either healthy or unhealthy.

The relationship between fats (triglycerides), cholesterol, and heart disease was originally presented in the "seven countries study." This study recommended that fat intake be reduced to 30 percent of total energy intake. However, the study revealed that in the Netherlands, the percentage of energy derived from fat was 48 percent, but the population's life expectancy was one of the highest in Europe! Similarly, in Crete, fat consumption was 40 percent of total energy intake, but the incidence of heart disease was one of the lowest in Europe. These inconsistencies have never been satisfactorily explained, although we agree that very high cholesterol levels (more than 300 mg/dL) are significantly related to coronary artery disease.[5]

Furthermore, the clinical studies directed at lowering blood lipids, including cholesterol, have shown no consistent decrease in death rates in spite of success in lowering cholesterol. In some studies more than half the patients with coronary disease had cholesterol levels below 200 mg/dL.[6] The message is in most instances that total cholesterol alone is not a reliable indicator for the risk of cardiovascular disease.

# 30 | Frequently Asked Questions

The following are questions that have been asked frequently since publication of the original *Sugar Busters! Cut Sugar to Trim Fat.*

Q1. Most doctors and nutritionists still say it is calories consumed versus calories burned that determines weight gain or loss. Why do you say otherwise, and what is your evidence?

A1. We say it is calories consumed versus calories *utilized* by the body. The body metabolizes the calories in some foods differently than in other foods. We have observed in ourselves and in others that the intake of low-glycemic carbohydrates or even calorie-dense meats or plant fats such as olive oil helps provide a greater long-term weight loss compared to lower total calorie intake of high-glycemic carbohydrates. Clinical trials have shown that the body mass index came out lower for subjects who were fed diets of equal calories but lower-glycemic-index carbohydrates.

Q2. How much protein is too much or dangerous?

A2. We find no research that shows that a diet of 30 percent protein is harmful except for people who have preexisting kidney disease. On the other hand, to eat 50 percent protein (plus the associated fat) means one would likely miss out on a sufficient quantity of vitamins, minerals, fiber, and other nutrients normally consumed in a diet with a higher percentage of fruits and vegetables.

Q3. Is whole milk unhealthy and will it make you gain weight?

A3. It is healthy and, consumed in the same quantity as skim milk, should not make you gain weight. Whole milk will, however, add to the total saturated fat in your diet if all other food consumption remains the same.

Q4. Which is healthier to eat, butter or margarine?

A4. Since many margarines still contain trans fats (the bad fats), we would say you would be safer choosing butter unless the margarine specifically says it contains no trans fats. However, unlike margarine, a very small quantity of salted butter can impart a flavor enhancement not achievable with margarines. By the way, if you use unsalted butter, you may inadvertently use a larger quantity while trying to achieve the same flavor enhancement.

Q5. Since fiber is not found in meats, will a diet of only 40 percent carbohydrate contain enough fiber?

A5. Yes, but only if the carbohydrates are (as recommended in *Sugar Busters!*) predominantly the low-glycemic-index, high-fiber kind.

Q6. How long can a person safely and successfully remain on the *Sugar Busters!* lifestyle?

A6. Forever!

# 31 | Sugar Busters! Products

In response to the many early and continuing requests we received to develop and offer products that would be acceptable for anyone following the *Sugar Busters!* lifestyle, we are now marketing a variety of foods in certain areas of the United States. To determine if the foods are available in your particular area, visit the new Web site at sugarbuster foods.com, which is controlled by the same people who market Camellia brand products, our new licensee, who oversee the manufacturing and distribution of the products. If the products are not available in your local supermarket, request that the store or area manager obtain the products.

There are other books now available that recommend the consumption of lower-glycemic-index foods. In our opinion, the line of products offered under the Author's Choice (*Sugar Busters!*) brand should be compatible on several of these diets such as *The Zone*, *Protein Power*, or even the later phases of the Atkins diet. Of course, beyond the diets just mentioned, we firmly believe these products would also be good for anyone interested in a healthy eating pattern. The products should be particularly useful to diabetics, who, once beginning a low-glycemic way of eating, will want to have their doctor monitor their new, lower medication requirements.

The following products are being manufactured as Sugar Busters!®, Author's Choice™ Brand Foods:

7 types of 100% whole-wheat, whole-grain breads, rolls and/or pita

6 types of 100% whole-wheat pastas

5 types of sugar-free salad dressings

1 type of sugar-free mayonnaise

6 flavors of no-sugar-added sports drinks (Refresher)

4 flavors of no-sugar-added ice cream

4 flavors of sugar-free pops (frozen ice bars)

6 flavors of no-sugar-added yogurts

# 32 | Sugar Busters!
##   | Support Groups

If you're reading *Sugar Busters!* you must be motivated to lose weight and/or improve your blood
chemistry. Your new knowledge changes your attitude about the way that you eat and what happens
when you eat. Can your initial motivation, attitude,
and success alone keep you from lapsing into your
old, fat-accumulating way of eating? For many of
you the answer is yes. For others, it is more difficult
to avoid the ever-present temptations to stray from
the new lifestyle. What can best fuel your persever-
ance? This chapter is for those who would like a
little help in not yielding to temptation.

Countless individuals have been able to lose
weight and remain at their desired weight by
following *Sugar Busters!* Others have found encouragement and support on the Sweettalk Plus Board of
the Sugar Busters Web site (www.sugarbusters.com),
which provides an online way to exchange ideas
on recipes, "legal" foods, and answers for specific
problems.

But what about the individuals who need even

more help? We think that a support group just might be the answer and we want to provide you with a plan for starting a support group and ideas to make it effective.

There are strong forces that work against our initial motivation. A holiday or family celebration can cause us to interrupt our dietary regimen. Other life events that factor into our failed attempts are family and relationship problems, difficulty at the job, hectic schedules, and even bouts with depression. We also may remember that we constantly experienced previous failures at dieting. Of course, we have been given the wrong information on how to lose weight: "lower your fat intake" rather than "choose the correct carbohydrates."

Why might you want to use a support group? A support group can help provide its members with an opportunity for mutual growth and change. Members share similar difficulties and feelings, offering a sense of "being in the same boat." The group affords members the experience of learning that others are facing the same troublesome problems. The exchange of knowledge and ideas will promote progress. Members can merge their goals with the optimistic goals of others in the group to move forward. A support group also provides encouragement when members encounter roadblocks, like the occasional plateaus (see Chapter 22), and offers different perspectives to success in meeting goals.

A support group can be as structured or as informal

as members desire. For example, two or more individuals can meet to walk together several times a week and talk about their progress on *Sugar Busters!* Or the support group can be a weekly or monthly meeting at a set location with several or many members, a designated leader, and a planned agenda. Either group can be tremendously successful for those involved.

Although there can be great flexibility in format, there are several time-tested rules that should be followed in any support group. One goal for the group should be to create a warm, nonjudgmental atmosphere so that members can feel free to talk without embarrassment. Derogatory comments should not be allowed.

**Confidentiality** must be respected to foster an atmosphere of trust among members. Keeping personal disclosures confidential is essential.

Avoid giving medical opinions. That advice should be left to the medical profession. Group members can, however, relate their own personal experiences of health improvement from the *Sugar Busters!* way of eating.

**Rotate group leadership.** Sharing in this task will give everyone a sense of belonging and participation. One of the most important roles of the group leader is to encourage participation by all members but, at the same time, not force anyone to share their personal experiences unless they feel comfortable doing so. The group leader should try to keep the discussions interesting and lively by not allowing anyone, including the leader, to dominate the conversation. A statement like "Let's hear from someone else about this topic" can be effective in moving the discussion along.

**To get started,** get the core organizers together and choose from the following suggestions and guidelines, taking time at the first meeting to decide on a preliminary format that can be fine-tuned at future meetings.

1. Choose a group leader and a group name, and discuss leader rotation.
2. Decide on how large you want the group to be and solicit members through friends, work, church, social groups, and exercise facilities.
3. Decide on a meeting place: members' homes, church, school, or library facilities.
4. Decide on the time and frequency of meetings.
5. Collect contact information: telephone numbers, home addresses, and e-mail addresses.
6. Discuss group policy such as confidentiality and respect for the opinion of others.
7. Decide on a format for meetings. Having a format will help to bring more ideas and topics for discussion.

The above guidelines usually enhance the effectiveness of most support groups. However, after business is taken care of, then it's time for encouragement, support, cohesion, and most of all progress to begin. Normally, the level of lively discussion and exchange of ideas will increase in future meetings. An important thing to remember is that you are not in the group to "fix" someone else. Rather, you are participating in the group to gain insight into your own behavior, receive and give feedback, support, knowledge, and encouragement to each other. We offer the following ideas for format and discussion to get you started.

Begin the first group discussion by asking members to briefly tell their story, but do not force anyone to talk until they feel comfortable in doing so.

Discuss how progress in weight loss will be discussed. Many individuals report three numbers: initial weight, current weight, and desired weight. Have a *Sugar Busters!* book available for reference at meetings.

Members should be encouraged to bring to the meeting articles on the health benefits of different fruits, vegetables, and grains, new ideas for discussion, product information; or recipes from the Sweet-talk Board. Bring seasonal *Sugar Busters!* recipes.

Compile a group list of precipitating events or feelings that coincided with overeating or "cheating." Patterns of behavior may begin to become evident. These psychological causes for eating problems can become an ongoing subject for discussion during group meetings.

If some members desire, initiate a buddy system so that members can call each other during the week if eating problems occur.

Limit refreshments to non-sugar-sweetened drinks. Occasionally, perhaps every other month, have a potluck supper with members bringing their favorite *Sugar Busters!* dish with copies of the recipe for all. Be sure to plan so that there is just enough food to go around—and remember, no second helpings except on green leafy salads.

The leader should prepare a short opening statement that can be used at the beginning of each meeting that will help members to reaffirm their commitment to the *Sugar Busters!* way of eating and their belief in the strength of the group endeavor. As improvements in weight and health become visible, the group will bond and become more of a team, and no one will want to let the team down by straying from his or her individual goals. This is a great motivational enhancement provided through group (team) dynamics. If some members are more competitive than others, let them simply exceed their previously stated goals.

Make no mistake—*Sugar Busters!* is a way of life that is also very healthy. This is precisely why so many who have tried *Sugar Busters!* stick with it regardless of whether or not they need to lose weight. On *Sugar Busters!* we feel better, and in the *Sugar Busters!* support group we feel better together!

# Notes

## Chapter 1: Introduction
1. *Billings Gazette*, Section C, page 1, October 23, 2002.
2. *ABC World News Tonight* with Peter Jennings broadcast, August 22, 2002.
3. Avery Comarow, "America's Best Hospitals, 2002," *US News and World Report*, (July 23, 2001).
4. Personal communication with Dr. Margaret Spitz, M.D., October 1998.
5. "Secrets of Successful Dieters," *Harvard Women's Health Watch*, (May 2002): 4.
6. Personal communication with Dr. Ann DeWees Allen, M.D., nutritionist for the Tampa Bay Buccaneers.

## Chapter 2: The Glycemic Index
1. C. L. Larsson and G. K. Johansson, "Dietary Intake and Nutritional Status of Young Vegans and Omnivores in Sweden," *American Journal of Clinical Nutrition* 76, no. 1 (July 2002): 1100–1106.
2. K. W. Heaton, et al., "Particle Size of Wheat, Maize, and Oat Test Meals: Effects on Plasma, Glucose, and Insulin Response and on the Rate of Starch Digestion in Vitro," *American Journal of Clinical Nutrition* 47 (1998): 675–682.

3. Jane Brody, "Fear Not That Carrot, Potato or Ear of Corn," *The New York Times,* (June 11, 2000): D8.
4. Janis Jibrin, R.D., "The Good Carbs," *Prevention,* (May 2001): 144.
5. Jennie Brand-Miller, et al, *The Glucose Revolution Life Plan* (Marlowe & Co., 2001).
6. "Glycemic Load, Diet, and Health," *Harvard Women's Health Watch,* (June 2001): 1-2.

## Chapter 5: Prevention

1. D. F. Williamson, "The Prevention of Obesity," 341, *New England Journal of Medicine,* (October 7, 1999): 1140-1141.
2. Associated Press, "Study Verifies Obesity Dangers," *Billings Gazette,* (October 7, 1999): 24.
3. T. T. Fung et al., "Whole-Grain Intake and the Risk of Type 2 Diabetes: A Prospective Study in Men," *American Journal of Clinical Nutrition* 76, no. 3 (September 2002): 535-540.
4. Personal communication with Dr. Paul K. Welton, M.D., M.Sc.
5. *Consumer Reports on Health,* (June 2002): 7.
6. "You've Survived the Cancer: Now What?" *Tufts University Health and Nutrition Letter,* (February 2003): 1.

## Chapter 6: The Epidemic of Childhood Obesity (and What to Do About It)

1. N. Pierce, "Physical Education Is Getting Set for a Comeback," *San Antonio Express,* (April 1, 2002).
2. L. Garcia, "Picking Up the Pace in PE: The Right Move?" *Dallas Morning News,* (May 10, 2002): 11A.
3. Nanci Hellmich, "Extra Weight Shaves Years Off Lives," *USA Today,* (January 7, 2003): 2A.

## Chapter 8: Insulin

1. C. R. Kahn and G. C. Weir, *Joslin's Diabetes Mellitus*, 13th ed. (Philadelphia: Lea and Febiger, 1994).
2. J. J. O'Keefe Jr., C. J. Lavie Jr., and B. D. McCallister, "Insights into the Pathogenesis and Prevention of Coronary Artery Disease," *Mayo Clinic Proceedings*, (1995) 70: 69-79.
3. T.M.S. Wolever, et al., "Beneficial Effects of Low-Glycemic Index Diet in Overweight NIDDM Subjects," *Diabetes Care*, (1992) 15: 562-64.
4. D.J.A. Jenkins, et al., "Glycemic Index of Foods: A Physiological Basis for Carbohydrate Exchange," *American Journal of Clinical Nutrition*, (1981) 34: 362-66.

## Chapter 11: Acceptable Foods and Substitutes

1. W. C. Knowler, et al., "Diabetes Mellitus in the Pima Indians: Incidence, Risk Factors amd Pathogenesis," *Diabetes and Metabolism Review*, (1990) 6: 1-27.

## Chapter 13: Why <u>Sugar Busters!</u> Works for Diabetics

1. "Experts Define 'Pre-Diabetes' and Call for Screening," *Tufts University Health and Nutrition Letter*, (May, 2002): 7.
2. W. C. Knowler, et al., "Diabetes Mellitus in the Pima Indians: Incidence, Risk Factors amd Pathogenesis," *Diabetes and Metabolism Review*, (1990) 6: 1-27.
3. Jennie B. Miller, et al., *The GI Factor* (Rydalmere, Australia: Hodder Headline Australia PTY Ltd., 1996).
4. Anita Manning, *USA Today*, (April 17, 2002).
5. "TV Watching and Diabetes," *Consumer Reports on Health*, (February 2002): 6.

6. *Journal of the American Medical Association,* (February 12, 1997) Vol. 277. No. 6.

## Chapter 15: **Sugar Busters!** for the Healthy Heart

1. A. C. Guyton and S. E. Hall, *Textbook of Medical Physiology,* 10th ed. (Philadelphia: W. B. Saunders, 2000).

## Chapter 17: Exercise

1. *Tufts Univerity Health and Nutrition Letter,* (July 2002): 6.

## Chapter 18: Super Foods

1. "Supplements Slow the Course of Macular Degeneration," *Harvard Women's Health Watch,* (December 2001): 1-2.
2. "Fruits and Veggies Protect Your Heart," *Environmental Nutrition,* (August 2002): 1.
3. "How Beans Help Your Heart," *Consumer Reports on Health,* (August 2002): 6.
4. "Say Nuts to Diabetes," *Massachusetts Medical Society Health News,* (February 2003): 4.
5. C. M. Albert et al., "Blood Levels of Long-Chain n-3 Fatty Acids and the Risk of Sudden Death," *New England Journal of Medicine* 346, no. 15 (April 11, 2002): 1113-1118.
6. "Bring on the Chocolates, Valentine!" *Harvard Women's Health Watch,* (February 2002)" 3.

## Chapter 19: Soft Drinks, Hard Facts

1. *Joint Report of the American Dental Association and the Council on Scientific Affairs to the House of Delegates: Response to Resolution 73 H-2000* (October 2001).
2. D. S. Ludwig et al., "Relation Between Consumption of Sugar-Sweetened Drinks and Childhood Obesity: A

Prospective, Observational Analysis," *The Lancet* 357, no. 9255, (February 17, 2001).

3. S. R. Williams, *Nutrition and Diet Therapy*, 11th ed. (St. Louis : Times Mirror/Mosby College Publishers, 2001).

4. G. Warshak, "Teenage Girls, Carbonated Beverages, and Bone Fractures," *Archives of Pediatric and Adolescent Medicine* 154, no. 6 (June 2000): 610-613.

5. Personal communication with Dr. Jim Landers, D.D.S.

## Chapter 25: To Drink or Not to Drink

1. "HowWine Took Center Stage," *Wine Spectator*, (December 15, 2001): 45.

2. Ibid.

3. Pat Hentik-Mansson, "Recommending Alcohol for the Elderly," *Wine Spectator*, (December 15, 2001): 62.

## Chapter 26: Fat Versus Low-Fat Diets and Products

1. Gary Taubes, "The Soft Science of Dietary Fat," *Science*, (March 2001): 2536-2545.

2. Nancy Hellmich, "Intake of Calories, Fat Up," *USA Today*, (January 17, 1996).

3. "Reduced Fat/Low Calorie," *Massachusetts Medical Society Health News*, (August 2002): 9.

4. "Most Feared Cancers: For Women, It's Breast Cancer. Can Diet Help?" *Environmental Nutrition*, (August 2002): 4.

## Chapter 29: Myths

1. P. Webb, "The Measurement of Energy Exchange in Man: An Analysis," *American Journal of Clinical Nutrition* 33, no. 6 (1980): 1299-1310.

2. R. Liebel et al., "Changes in Energy Expenditure Resulting from Altered Body Weight," *New England Journal of Medicine* 322 (1995):621.

3. J. J. O'Keefe Jr., C. J. Lavie Jr., and B. D. McCallister, "Insight into the Pathogenesis and Prevention of Coronary Artery Disease," *Mayo Clinic Proceedings* (1995) 70: 69-79.

4. M. deLorgeril, N. Manelle, and P. A. Salen, "A Mediterranean Type Diet in the Secondary Prevention of Coronary Artery Disease," *Circulation* 88 (Suppl.) (1993): 1-165.

5. S. M. Artaude-Wild, et al., "Differences in Coronary Mortality Can Be Explained by Differences in Cholesterol and Saturated Fat Intakes in 40 Countries but Not in France and Finland: A Paradox," *Circulation* 88 (1993): 2771-2779.

6. K. M. Anderson, W. P. Castelli, and D. Levy, "Cholesterol and Mortality: 30 Years of Follow-Up from the Framingham Study," *Journal of the American Medical Association* 257 (1987): 2176-2180.

# Glossary

**Amino acids**   the building blocks of all protein. There are nine essential, or necessary, amino acids that the body cannot make itself and that must be provided from the foods we eat (an egg contains all nine).

**Amylase**   enzymes secreted by the salivary glands and the pancreas that break down carbohydrates.

**Antioxidants**   chemical compounds that readily accept an oxygen-free radical, thus inhibiting the oxidation of polyunsaturated fatty acids that are important to maintaining cellular health. Vitamins A, C, and E are antioxidants.

**Atheroma**   (also referred to as a *plaque*) a deposit of cholesterol, calcium, and blood clot in the lining of major vessels, eventually leading to blockage.

**Arteriosclerosis**   the process of hardening of arteries through the formation of plaques on the inner lining of major blood vessels.

**Beta cells**   specialized cells in the pancreas responsible for the production and secretion of insulin.

**Bioflavonoids**   compounds found in nature mostly as yellow pigments that contain no nutritional value, but may help preserve the health of arterial walls by reducing their cholesterol content.

**Blood clot**   coagulated or congealed blood.

**Calorie**   The unit of heat energy required to raise 1 kilogram of water 1 degree Celsius.

**Carbohydrates**   chemical compounds containing carbon, hydrogen, and oxygen. Carbohydrates are a storage form of sugar.

**Cholesterol**   a compound belonging to a family of substances called sterols. It usually combines with fat when circulating in the bloodstream for distribution to all cells.

**Complex carbohydrate**   a carbohydrate with a more complex structure, such as starch or glycogen. The degree of complexity does not indicate the rate at which the carbohydrate is digested.

**Dextrose**   a sugar which is chemically identical to glucose.

**Diabetes mellitus, Type 1**   a disease characterized by the lack of insulin and resulting in elevated blood glucose (sugar) levels.

**Diabetes mellitus, Type 2**   a disease characterized by resistance of the cells in the body to the actions of insulin and that also leads to elevated blood glucose (sugar) levels.

**Energy**   capacity to produce motion or heat.

**Free fatty acid**   the structural component of fat.

**Fructose**   a simple sugar found in fruits. Its insulin-stimulating effect is lower than that of galactose and glucose.

**Galactose** a simple sugar found in dairy products. Its insulin-stimulating effect is less than glucose.

**Gastric emptying** the process of emptying food from the stomach or the time required to empty a meal from the stomach.

**Glucagon** hormone secreted by the pancreas that helps regulate blood sugar and metabolize stored fat.

**Glucose** the form in which sugar circulates in the bloodstream; the body's main energy source.

**Glycemic index** how rapidly a carbohydrate food is digested into glucose and how much it causes the blood sugar (glucose) to rise.

**Glyceride** a group name for fats. Mono-, di-, and triglycerides, which contain one, two, or three fatty acids, are the main constituents of fats.

**Glycerol** a constituent of fats. Chemically, it is an alcohol that combines with fatty acids to produce fats.

**Glycerol-3-phosphate** a metabolic product that occurs when glucose transforms into triglycerides.

**Glycogen** a complex form of glucose that is stored in the liver and muscle to be used to meet energy needs.

**High-density lipoprotein (HDL)** lipoproteins carrying cholesterol from the cells to the liver for breakdown and elimination from the body, probably the single best determinant of risk for coronary artery disease and heart attacks.

**High-density lipoprotein (HDL) cholesterol** high-density lipoprotein cholesterol thought to be protective against heart disease.

**Hyperglycemia** abnormally elevated blood glucose (sugar) level.

**Hyperlipidemia** abnormally elevated blood lipids, usually either cholesterol or triglycerides or both.

**Hypertension** persistently elevated blood pressure.

**Hypoglycemia** an abnormally low blood glucose (sugar) level.

**Insulin** hormone secreted by the pancreas. It lowers blood glucose by directing cells to utilize the glucose.

**Insulin resistance** failure of insulin to exert its normal effect of allowing glucose into cells. This causes a rise in blood glucose (sugar) levels and therefore triggers the need for still more insulin.

**Lipase** enzymes secreted by the pancreas that help digest fats.

**Lipid** a fat of either plant or animal origin.

**Lipogenesis** the formation of fat from glucose.

**Lipolysis** the breakdown of triglycerides to free fatty acids and glycerol, both of which are used as energy sources for the body.

**Lipoproteins** combination of fat and proteins that circulate in the bloodstream. They function as the major carriers of lipids.

**Lipoprotein lipase** a very important enzyme in the storage of fat.

**Liver** a large organ that directs the metabolism of carbohydrates, proteins, and fats and the manufacture of enzymes, cholesterol, and other important substances. Our "metabolic computer."

**Low-density lipoproteins (LDL)** lipoproteins that are important in the transport of cholesterol.

**Low-density lipoprotein (LDL) cholesterol** low-density lipoprotein cholesterol, thought to be a major risk factor for heart disease.

**Lymphatic system** small vessels that drain tissue fluid back into the cardiovascular system. It is the main route of absorption of fats from the small intestine.

**Maltose** A disaccharide composed of two molecules of glucose. It is the fundamental structural unit of glycogen and starch.

**Metabolism** the sum of all the chemical and physiological processes by which the body grows and maintains itself and by which it breaks matter down into a new state.

**Modulate** regulate or control the flow of.

**Monounsaturated fats** fat molecules containing only one double bond. Examples are the oils found in olives, peanuts, and pecans.

**Obesity** the presence of excess body fat.

**Osteoporosis** loss of bone mass that often leads to fractures.

**Pancreas** an important organ that produces both insulin and glucagon, as well as digestive enzymes such as lipase.

**Phytochemicals** chemicals and nutrients that are derived from plants.

**Plasma fibrinogen** protein used in making blood clots.

**Plaque**  deposits of cholesterol, calcium, and blood clot on the lining of major vessels. Also called *atheroma*.

**Platelets**  elements in blood that are important in the clotting process by sticking to each other and starting the process of clot formation.

**Polyunsaturated fats**  fat molecules containing two or more double bonds. Most vegetable oils are polyunsaturated.

**Saturated fats**  fat molecules containing carbon atoms that are fully bound with hydrogen atoms, found in most animal fats.

**Simple sugars**  also known as *monosaccharides*. The most important are glucose, fructose (fruit sugar), and galactose (milk sugar).

**Sleep apnea**  diminished respiration during sleep; often associated with obesity.

**Sterols**  complex steroids, one of which is cholesterol.

**Syndrome X**  the combination of two or more of the following: insulin resistance, elevated insulin levels, elevated triglycerides, obesity, and hypertension.

**Synthesis**  the manufacture or creation of a new substance.

**Trans fats**  fats similar to saturated fats, which can be produced by heating oil; trans fats increase LDL (bad cholesterol) and reduce HDL (good cholesterol).

**Triglycerides**  the main type of stored fat in most animal systems.

**Type 1 diabetes mellitus**  a disease characterized by the lack of insulin and the resulting elevated blood glucose (sugar) levels.

**Type 2 diabetes mellitus**  a disease characterized by resistance of the cells in the body to the actions of insulin and that also leads to elevated blood glucose (sugar) levels.

**Very low density lipoproteins (VLDL)**  lipoproteins that are important in transport of fatty components from the liver to fat cells.

# Appendix A

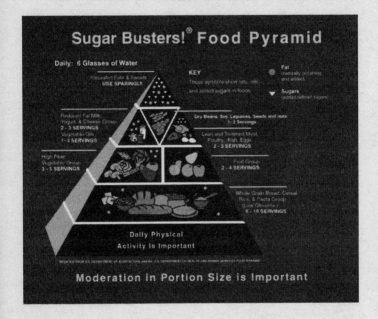

# Index

# Permissions Acknowledgments

Grateful acknowledgment is made to the following for permission to reprint previously published recipes:

Rick Bayless: "Ceviche Clasico," "Mexican Beans," and "Grilled Salmon with Lemon-and-Thyme Scented Salsa Veracruzana" from *Mexico: One Plate at a Time* by Rick Bayless. Copyright © 2000 by Rick Bayless. Reprinted by permission of Rick Bayless, Scribner, an imprint of Simon & Schuster Adult Publishing Group, and The Doe Coover Agency.

Tom Douglas: "Tom's Tasty Sashimi Tuna Salad with Whole Wheat Green Onion Pancakes" and "Sake Sauce" from *TOM DOUGLAS' SEATTLE KITCHEN* by Tom Douglas. Copyright © 2001 by Tom Douglas. Reprinted by permission of Tom Douglas and William Morrow, an imprint of HarperCollins Publishers, Inc.

Daniel Orr: "Herb Perfumed Chicken Breast with Vegetable Fleurettes and Sweet Potatoes," "Master Blend: Mixed Peppers (Aux Poivres)," "Tuna Steak Aux Poivres," and "Barley Salad with Chili, Herb, and Lime Vinaigrette" from *DANIEL ORR REAL FOOD* by Daniel Orr. Copyright © 1997 by Daniel Orr. Reprinted by permission of Daniel Orr and Rizzoli International Publications.

Grateful acknowledgment is given to the chefs and restaurants listed below for their generosity in offering recipes for *The New Sugar Busters!*

Mark Abernathy of Loca Luna (Little Rock, AR); Rick Bayless of Topolobampo (Chicago, IL); Franklin Becker of Capitale (New York, NY); Jesse Cool of Flea Street Café (Menlo Park, CA); Gary Coyle of Tavern on the Green (New York, NY); Sheri Davis of Dish (Atlanta, GA); Tom Douglas of Dahlia Lounge (Seattle, WA); Jean-Marie Dubos of Hotel Crescent Court (Dallas, TX); Dean Fearing of the Mansion on Turtle Creek (Dallas, TX); Susanna Foo of Susanna Foo Chinese Cuisine (Philadelphia, PA); Dominic Galati of Dominic's (St. Louis, MO); Gilbert Garza of Suze (Dallas, TX); Bernard Guillas of The Marine Room (La Jolla, CA); Ray Henry of Caneel Bay (St. John, US Virgin Islands); Shoji Hirota of Hotel Seiyo Ginza (Tokyo, Japan); Chris Janssens of The Dharmawangsa (Jakarta, Indonesia); Aaron Keller of Humpy's Great Alaskan Alehouse (Anchorage, AK); Roxanne Klein of Roxanne's (Larkspur, CA); Deborah Knight of Mosaic (Scottsdale, AZ); Marc Lippman of Las Ventanas al Paraiso (Baja California Sur, Mexico); Tim Love of The Lonesome Dove Western Bistro (Fort Worth, TX); Tory McPhail of Commander's Palace (New Orleans, LA); Johnny and Mary Jo Mosca of Mosca's Restaurant (Avondale, LA); Eberhard Mueller of Bayard's (New York, NY); Daniel Orr of Guastavino's (New York, NY); Warren Pearson of Al Faisaliah (Riyadh, Saudi Arabia); Francis Perrin of Frederick's (San Antonio, TX); Milton Prudence of Galatoire's (New Orleans, LA); Patricia Radicevic of Three Brothers Restaurant (Milwaukee, WI); Tom Rapp of Etats-Unis (New York, NY); Michael Reuter of Little Dix Bay (Virgin Gorda, the British Virgin Islands); Michael Richard of Citronelle (Washington DC); Hans Röckenwagner of Röckenwagner (Santa Monica, CA); Charlie Socher of Café Matou (Chicago, IL); Tony Vallone of Tony's (Houston, TX); Bob Waggoner of Charleston Grill (Charleston, SC)

# About the Authors

**H. Leighton Steward** has a master of science degree from Southern Methodist University and became CEO of a Fortune 500 energy company. He also authored a booklet on causes of land loss of the lower Mississippi River wetland system. One hundred thousand of these booklets are in circulation worldwide and are referred to by many educational and governmental institutions. He is on the boards of the M. D. Anderson Cancer Center in Houston, Texas, and Tulane University in New Orleans and is chairman of the board of trustees at the Institute for the Study of Earth and Man (anthropology, geology, and statistics) at SMU in Dallas, Texas, and is immediate past chairman of the Audubon Nature Institute in New Orleans. His own success with this way of eating and a family history of diabetes motivated him to write *SUGAR BUSTERS!®*.

**Morrison C. Bethea, M.D.,** is a graduate of Davidson College and Tulane University School of Medicine. He completed his postgraduate training in thoracic and cardiac surgery at Columbia-Presbyterian Medical Center in New York. Currently he practices thoracic, cardiac, and vascular surgery in New Orleans. He is the medical consultant to Freeport-McMoRan, Inc., and sits on the board of McMoRan Exploration Co. and Tenet's Memorial Medical Center of New Orleans. Dr Bethea is a diplomate of the American Board of Thoracic Surgery, a clinical professor of surgery at Tulane Medical Center, and an author of many publications in the field of cardiovascular disease.

**Samuel S. Andrews, M.D.,** is a graduate of Louisiana State University School of Medicine. He is a recognized expert in the treatment of obesity, and practices endocrinology with the Audubon Internal Medicine Group. Dr. Andrews has authored several scientific publications and is currently conducting nutrional low-glycemic carbohydrate research studies in both adults and children. He is a fellow in the American College of Physicians and the American College of Endocrinology. He is a clinical associate professor of medicine at the Louisiana State University Medical School in New Orleans and a member of the Louisiana State University Medical Center Pancreatic Transplant Team.

**Luis A. Balart, M.D.,** is a graduate of Louisiana State University School of Medicine. He completed his training in gastroenterology at the Ochsner Clinic and in hepatology at the University of Southern California. Dr. Balart is the chief of gastroenterology at the LSU School of Medicine in New Orleans and is Medical Director of Liver Transplantation at Memorial Medical Center. He is actively involved in ongoing clinical trials in the treatment of chronic viral hepatitis and chronic liver disorders. He is the author of many publications in these areas.